IMMUNOLOGY AND IMMUNE SYSTEM DISORDERS

TH17 CELLS IN HEALTH AND DISEASE

IMMUNOLOGY AND IMMUNE SYSTEM DISORDERS

Additional books and e-books in this series can be found on Nova's website under the Series tab.

This book is dedicated to all my colleagues that help me in my practice, to my family and my patients.

CONTENTS

Preface		**ix**
Chapter 1	Th17 Cells in Health *Tsvetelina Velikova*	**1**
Chapter 2	The Role of Th17 Cells in Osteoclastogenesis and Rheumatoid Arthritis *Yuki Nanke and Shigeru Kotake*	**11**
Chapter 3	Phenotypic and Functional Heterogeneity of Th17 Cells in Systemic Sclerosis *Rositsa V. Karalilova*	**31**
Chapter 4	The Role of Th17 Cells in Spondyloarthritis *Yuki Nanke and Shigeru Kotake*	**61**
Chapter 5	Allergic Rhinitis, IL-17 and the Concept of a Common Respiratory Pathway *Kremena Naydenova, Tsvetelina Velikova* *and Vasil Dimitrov*	**83**
Chapter 6	Th17 Cells in Childhood Asthma *Snezhina Lazova, Guergana Petrova* *and Tsvetelina Velikova*	**99**

viii   *Contents*

Chapter 7   Th17 Cells and Cystic Fibrosis   **115**
                   Guergana Petrova, Snezhina Lazova
                   and Tsvetelina Velikova

Chapter 8   Multiple Sclerosis: Th17 Cells in
                   Immunopathogenesis and Therapy   **137**
                   Marina Ivanova, Ivan Milanov,
                   Ekaterina Krasimirova, Dobroslav Kyurkchiev
                   and Tsvetelina Velikova

Chapter 9   Inflammatory Bowel Disease in Children and
                   Adolescents: Th17 Cells and Other Players   **151**
                   Rayna R. Shentova-Eneva

Chapter 10   Th17/Tregs Cells in Patients with Ulcerative
                   Colitis during Anti-TNFα Therapy   **171**
                   Tsvetelina Velikova, Ekaterina Ivanova-Todorova,
                   Zoya Spasova, Maria Petkova,
                   Ekaterina Krasimirova,
                   Kalina Tumangelova-Yuzeir, Georgi Vasilev,
                   Lyudmila Mateva and Dobroslav Kyurkchiev

Chapter 11   Th17 Cells Involvement in Celiac Disease   **187**
                   Gergana Taneva and Tsvetelina Velikova

Chapter 12   Th17 Cells and Other Pathologies   **205**
                   Tsvetelina Velikova

Chapter 13   The Controversial Interaction between Th17
                   and T Regulatory Cells in Autoimmunity   **221**
                   Tsvetelina Velikova

About the Editor   **231**

Index   **233**

Related Nova Publications   **245**

PREFACE

Although described more than ten years ago, Th17 cells are still a focus of interest and investigation, as well as a source of passionate debating and controversial potential for future therapeutic approaches.

These cells play an essential role in protective immunity, especially on mucosal surfaces, but also contribute to chronic inflammation in autoimmune disorders. There is still lack of understanding of how Th17 cells transform from non-pathogenic to the major pathological players in the organism.

The pathogenesis of many inflammatory, allergic, autoimmune, and tumor disorders are assumed to depend on activated Th17 cells and their related cytokines. The role of IL-17 and Th17 in different pathways has also changed the perspective of immunology regarding the basis of chronic tissue inflammation. The existing concepts of immunopathologic mechanisms related to Th17 cells in various pathological processes are extended further in the last decades and have been supported by many studies.

Furthermore, the number of conditions influenced by Th17 cells seems to increase. However, in most of them, the exact mechanisms of action of Th17 cells remain unclear, though evidence suggests that they could also play an essential role in the control of these diseases.

Moreover, the described conversion between Th17 and Treg cells makes the picture more complicated and confusing. Regulation of this balance, as well as the control of Th17-mediated inflammation, are the main elements in the development of therapeutic strategies for some immune-mediated diseases.

In: Th17 Cells in Health and Disease
Editor: Tsvetelina Velikova

ISBN: 978-1-53617-152-5
© 2020 Nova Science Publishers, Inc.

Chapter 1

TH17 CELLS IN HEALTH

Tsvetelina Velikova, MD, PhD*
Clinical Immunology, University Hospital Lozenetz,
Sofia University, Sofia, Bulgaria

ABSTRACT

Th17 cells are CD4+ effector T lymphocytes, mainly characterized by the secretion of IL-17 cytokine, that play an essential role in immunity, especially on mucosal surfaces, but also contribute to chronic inflammation in autoimmune disorders. However, the presence of Th17 lymphocytes is not always pathological, although they are categorized as pro-inflammatory. Th17 cells also protect against extracellular bacteria such as Streptococcus pneumoniae. Different cell types other than Th17 cells can secrete IL-17A, including gdT cells, innate lymphoid cells, B cells and T regulatory cells, but it is still unclear how different cell sources of the cytokine contribute to the host protection.

There is still lack of understanding of how Th17 cells transform from non-pathogenic and even protective lymphocytes to the major pathological players in the disease. Approaches that efficiently alter Th17 immunity will be significant to accelerate vaccine and drug development programs.

---

* Corresponding Author's Email: tsvelikova@medfac.mu-sofia.bg.

Keywords: Th17 cells, IL-17, CD4+ T lymphocytes, T regulatory cells, mucosa, pneumococci, vaccine, surface protection

INTRODUCTION

Th17 cells are CD4+ effector T lymphocytes, mainly characterized by the secretion of IL-17 cytokine (primarily IL-17A and IL-17F). They can also produce IL-22, IL-21, IL-10, IFNγ, and GM-CSF [1]. Th17 cells play an essential role in maintaining immunity, especially on mucosal surfaces, but also contribute to chronic inflammation in autoimmune disorders [3]. Although there are many studies on the role of Th17 cells in the pathogenesis of autoimmune and inflammatory diseases using animal models, clinical trials with agents against IL-17, and GWAS data, there is still lack of understanding of how Th17 cells transform from non-pathogenic and even protective lymphocytes to the major pathological players in the organism.

Phenotyping by flow cytometry showed that human Th17 cells possess a heterogeneous phenotype [3]. This observation was supported by studies on murine Th17 cells that revealed the existence of significant heterogeneity and clearly expressed Th17 cell subtypes at different stages of differentiation [4]. It is interesting to note that the immature Th17 cells have gene signatures similar to stem these cells. However, they usually reside in the lymph nodes. The mature Th17 cells have been identified as expressing high levels of Stat3 and RANK-L. Moreover, some of these mature subsets were shown to produce IFNγ [4].

Therefore, although Th17 cells are categorized as pro-inflammatory due to their production of IL-17, the presence of Th17 lymphocytes in the skin, colon, lungs, and tonsils, is not always pathological. Contrariwise, Th17 cells are involved in the protection of all mucosal surfaces and other tissues and organs in the body.

TH17 CELLS AND PROTECTION AGAINST INFECTIOUS AGENTS

It was shown that different pathogens induce diverse cytokine responses from Th17 cells. For example, Th17 cells induced by Candida albicans tend to produce IFNγ, whereas Th17 cells triggered by S. aureus are more likely to produce IL-10 [5]. The reason for that is because the transcriptional activity of Th17 cells depends on the exposure to pathogens. In the presence of IL-23 RUNX1 expression is enhanced, which leads to Th17 differentiation, whereas IL-12 alters T-bet expression with an expansion of Th1-like cells that produce mainly IFNγ [6].

Further studies have shown that mouse Th17 cells in the intestinal mucosa can be transdifferentiated to IL-10-producing regulatory T cells (Tr-1 cells). This process was shown to depend on the presence of aryl hydrocarbon receptor and TGFβ [1]. After treatment with TNFα inhibitors, IL-10-producing Th17 cells were also described [7].

However, earlier studies suggest that Th17 cells and Tregs were mutually exclusive. These studies indicated that Th17 cell differentiation might be inhibited by IL-2 and activation of STAT5. As we mentioned above, Th17 cells can be transdifferentiated to Tregs and vice versa, under the influence of the inflammatory milieu [8, 9].

In mice, Th17 cells can be transdifferentiated to T follicular helper (Tfh) cells in the Peyer patches. They can also promote the production of IgA from B cells [10]. In contrast, in an inflammatory medium containing IL-23, B lymphocyte-induced maturation protein-1 (Blimp-1) is induced. This binds to and suppresses the Bcl6 gene that is required for the development of Tfh, thus, promotes the emergence of a pathogenic Th17 phenotype [11].

PROTECTIVE ROLE OF TH17 AGAINST STREPTOCOCCAL PNEUMONIA INFECTION

There are enough studies that declare the pathogenic properties of Th17 cells. However, not all actions of Th17 cells are harmful - they also carry out protection against extracellular bacteria such as Streptococcus pneumoniae.

The gram-positive bacterium S. pneumoniae (pneumococci) causes significant morbidity and mortality in children under the age of five worldwide through a range of diseases, including meningitis, bacteremia, and pneumonia [12]. The importance of Th17 cells in protecting against mucosal pneumococcal infections has become increasingly recognized. Many studies support the critical role of Th17 responses in the prevention or reduction of pneumococcal diseases in mice models and humans [13]. The secreted inflammatory cytokine IL-17 is essential for the recruitment and activation of macrophages, monocytes, and neutrophils to the nasopharynx and other sites of inflammation, which are responsible for the clearance of this microorganism in the host [14].

Th17-mediated immunity is emerging as a critical factor in protection against the usually asymptomatic nasopharyngeal colonization, which is considered the first step in the pathogenesis of the disease. Colonization triggers an inflammatory response that, when unregulated, can lead to excessive mucosal damage, distributing to other host sites, and facilitating transmission between individuals [14]. Besides, previous colonization elicits both systemic IgG and pulmonary IL-17A production that reduce the duration of subsequent transportation events and inhibit the development of invasive pneumococcal infection, whereas the protection against lung infection is lost in the absence of CD4+ T cells or IL-17 [15]. Importantly, Th17 responses are critical against lung infection, while antibodies against invasive disease are required [15]. However, based on IL-17 protection against pneumococcal infections appears to be reduced or lost after a viral infection such as influenza [16]. The proposed explanation for this is viral regulation of interferon signaling, which in turn negatively regulates IL-17 responses to bacterial infections [16]. Therefore, an important avenue for future research is how IL-17A responses can be modulated in the presence of viral infections, especially in influenza or respiratory syncytial virus.

The defensive role of IL-17 in humans was also demonstrated by the following results. It was shown that IL-17 is produced after in vitro stimulation of the tonsils and peripheral blood mononuclear cells (PBMCs) with pneumococcal antigens (i.e., pneumolysin and whole-cell antigen) [13]. The most protective effect of IL-17 is enhanced opsonophagocytic killing of pneumococci by human neutrophil observed when the antibodies and complement are lacking together with the absence of IL-17A [13].

Moreover, Hoe et al., and other groups, have shown that high concentrations of IL-17 are associated with low pneumococcal nasal density in mice and children [13]. It was recently discovered that mucosal Tregs isolated from children with pneumococcal carriage are more numerous than in children without pneumococcal carriage [17]. These Tregs are also able to inhibit CD4+ T cell proliferation [17]. It was further demonstrated that stimulation with a pneumococcal whole-cell antigen induces the spread of Tregs and the production of IL-10 but not IL-17. These results in the nasal lymphoid tissue were not surprising, taking into account that the amounts of Th17 and Treg are inversely related.

On the contrary, mice that are resistant to pneumococcal pneumonia have significantly higher Tregs in their lungs than mice with invasive pneumonia, which is mediated by TGFb signaling [17]. This data verifies that the Th17/Treg balance is critical for the control of pneumococcal colonization and invasive disease. More studies in humans are needed to confirm these effects of both Th17 cells and Tregs during pneumococcal infection.

This consideration of IL-17 responses as critical for the protection against pneumococcal infection and has led to significant efforts to develop effective vaccines to improve immunity against pneumococci. Over the last decade, pneumococcal whole-cell vaccine (WCV) has entered Phase I and Phase II clinical trials in Indonesia and Kenya after being demonstrated that it can specifically induce IL-17 immune responses and prevent pneumococcal infections in mice [18]. This vaccine is based on a non-

6 *Tsvetelina Velikova*

encapsulated strain of S. pneumoniae and, unlike the current pneumococcal conjugate vaccines, presenting more benefits for humans by providing independent serotype protection [18]. The hope is that this nex-generation vaccine will change the current pneumococcus prevention strategies.

OTHER SOURCES OF IL-17 UNLIKE TH-17 CELLS FOR PROTECTION IN THE ORGANISM

Different cell types other than Th17, including gdT cells and innate lymphoid cells (ILC), can produce IL-17 for protection [19]. IL-17-producing gdT cells in the oral cavity are essential for the control of Candida infection. During influenza viral infection, IL-17 is secreted by gdT cells but not Th17 cells, suggesting different pathways of IL-17 regulation via IL-21R signaling [20]. In pneumococcal infection, IL-17 produced by both gdT cells and B cells participate in the experimentally mediated protection supporting the claim that other sources of IL-17 may be equally important in protecting the host from bacterial disease. However, gd-IL-17-mediated pathology was observed; thus, a rigorous safety study of potential new therapies aimed at enhancing IL-17 responses is needed [13].

Interestingly, ILCs also mediate the protection of fungal infection through IL-17 production in mice in an IL-23 dependent manner [20]. Recent studies also showed that B cells could produce IL-17 and provide protection during infection with Trypanosoma cruzi [13]. Similar mechanisms are observed in autoimmune diseases, such as rheumatoid arthritis, where IL-17-secreting B cells, NK, and CD14+ cells were described [22], suggesting that various cell types could be the source of IL-17.

There is also some evidence that Foxp3+Treg cells can differentiate into pathogenic Th17 cells in the presence of IL-6 or TNF-α [13]. New insights on the role of mucous membranes

However, further studies are required to clarify the different functions of these subsets as sources of IL-17 during infection.

THE THERAPEUTIC POTENTIAL OF THE IL-17-DRIVEN PROTECTIVE IMMUNITY

The manipulation of the Th17 cell to obtain protection or disease control require considerable research and clinical trials. This is especially true for the development of new vaccines and targeted therapists.

There is a need for new approaches and methods to refine the understanding of how Th17 responses can be promoted during infection or inhibited in the context of autoimmune diseases.

Talking for the pneumococcal disease and vaccines, it is still unclear whether different cell types sources of IL-17 determine different responses to the distinct immunological compartments in the host (e.g., blood, mucosal surfaces). If we apply such technologies to identify individual immune responses to vaccine or treatment, this will allow for forecasting the lack of response or poor treatment outcomes. In line with this, strategies that effectively modulate Th17 immunity will be critically important to accelerate vaccine and drug development programs.

CONCLUSION

Our knowledge of the role of the Th17 response in both protective and pathogenic immunity has increased significantly over the last decade. Mechanisms involved in the stimulation or inhibition of IL-17 secretion, as well as the documentation of other cell sources of IL-17, unlike Th17 cells, will allow development of next-generation therapies for several autoimmune, inflammatory, infectious, allergic or tumor diseases.

Future research using advanced technologies, such as omics tools, will make possible to focus on exploring more deeply the complex pathways and immune networks involved Th17 responses in humans, and to develop novel vaccines or drugs that modify Th17/Treg axis in health and disease.

REFERENCES

[1] Bystrom J, Clanchy FIL, Taher TE, et al. Functional and phenotypic heterogeneity of Th17 cells in health and disease. *Eur. J. Clin. Invest.* 2019;49(1):e13032.

[2] Stockinger B, Omenetti S. The dichotomous nature of T helper 17 cells. *Nat. Rev. Immunol.* 2017;17:535-544.

[3] Wong MT, Ong DE, Lim FS, et al. A high-dimensional atlas of human T cell diversity reveals tissue-specific trafficking and cytokine signatures. *Immunity.* 2016;45:442-456.

[4] Gaublomme JT, Yosef N, Lee Y, et al. Single-cell genomics unveils critical regulators of Th17 cell pathogenicity. *Cell.* 2015;163:1400-1412.

[5] Zielinski CE, Mele F, Aschenbrenner D, et al. Pathogen-induced human TH17 cells produce IFN-gamma or IL-10 and are regulated by IL-1beta. *Nature.* 2012;484:514-518.

[6] Wang Y, Godec J, Ben-Aissa K, et al. The transcription factors T-bet and Runx are required for the ontogeny of pathogenic interferon-gamma-producing T helper 17 cells. *Immunity.* 2014;40: 355-366.

[7] Evans HG, Roostalu U, Walter GJ, et al. TNF-alpha blockade induces IL-10 expression in human CD4 + T cells. *Nat. Commun.* 2014;5:3199.

[8] Laurence A, Tato CM, Davidson TS, et al. Interleukin-2 signaling via STAT5 constrains T helper 17 cell generation. *Immunity.* 2007;26:371-381.

[9] Komatsu N, Okamoto K, Sawa S, et al. Pathogenic conversion of Foxp3 + T cells into TH17 cells in autoimmune arthritis. *Nat. Med.* 2014;20:62-68.

[10] Hirota K, Turner JE, Villa M, et al. Plasticity of TH17 cells in Peyer's patches is responsible for the induction of T cell-dependent IgA responses. *Nat. Immunol.* 2013;14:372-379.

[11] Jain R, Chen Y, Kanno Y, et al. Interleukin-23-induced transcription factor Blimp-1 promotes pathogenicity of T helper 17 cells. *Immunity.* 2016;44:131-142.

[12] Lundgren A, Bhuiyan TR, et al. Characterization of Th17 responses to Streptococcus pneumoniae in humans: Comparisons between adults and children in a developed and a developing country. *Vaccine* 2012;30: 3897-907.

[13] Hoe E, Anderson J, Nathanielsz J, et al. The contrasting roles of Th17 immunity in human health and disease. *Microbiol. Immunol.* 2017;61(2):49-56.

[14] Marques J.M., Rial A., Munoz N., et al. Protection against Streptococcus pneumoniae serotype 1 acute infection shows a signature of Th17- and IFN-gammamediated immunity. *Immunobiology* 2012;217: 420-9.

[15] Cohen JM, Khandavilli S, Camberlein E, et al. (2011) Protective contributions against invasive Streptococcus pneumoniae pneumonia of antibody and Th17-cell responses to nasopharyngeal colonisation. *PLoS ONE* 6, 2011: e25558.

[16] Robinson KM, Kolls JK, Alcorn JF. The immunology of influenza virus-associated bacterial pneumonia. *Curr. Opin.* 2015; *Immunol.* 34: 59-67.

[17] Neill DR, Fernandes VE, Wisby L, et al. T regulatory cells control susceptibility to invasive pneumococcal pneumonia in mice. *PLoS Pathog.* 2012;8:e1002660.

[18] Alderson MR. Status of research and development of pediatric vaccines for Streptococcus pneumoniae. *Vaccine* 2016;34:2959-61.

[19] Sutton CE, Mielke LA, Mills KH. IL-17-producing gammadelta T cells and innate lymphoid cells. *Eur. J. Immunol.* 2012;42: 2221-31.

[20] Moser EK, Sun J, Kim TS, Braciale TJ. IL-21R signaling suppresses IL-17 gamma delta T cell responses and production of IL-17 related

cytokines in the lung at steady state and after Influenza A virus infection. *PLoS ONE* 2015;10: e0120169.

[21] Gladiator A, Wangler N, Trautwein-Weidner K, et al. Cutting edge: IL-17-secreting innate lymphoid cells are essential for host defense against fungal infection. *J. Immunol.* 2013;190: 521-5.

[22] Schlegel PM, Steiert I, Kotter I, Muller CA. B cells contribute to heterogeneity of IL-17 producing cells in rheumatoid arthritis and healthy controls. *PLoS ONE* 2013;8:e82580.

In: Th17 Cells in Health and Disease
Editor: Tsvetelina Velikova

ISBN: 978-1-53617-152-5
© 2020 Nova Science Publishers, Inc.

Chapter 2

THE ROLE OF TH17 CELLS IN OSTEOCLASTOGENESIS AND RHEUMATOID ARTHRITIS

Yuki Nanke[1,], MD, PhD and Shigeru Kotake[2], MD, PhD*

[1]Institute of Rheumatology,
Tokyo Women's Medical University, Tokyo, Japan
[2]Division of Rheumatology, First Department of Comprehensive
Medicine, Jichi Medical University Saitama Medical Center,
Saitama, Japan

ABSTRACT

Rheumatoid arthritis (RA) is a chronic inflammatory disease associated with synovitis and bone destruction. Monocyte/macrophage-derived cytokines, including tumor necrosis factor-alpha (TNF-α), interleukin-1 (IL-1), and IL-6, and T-cell-derived cytokine, IL-17, are involved in the pathogenesis of RA. In the study of human disease, it is

---

* Corresponding Author's Email: ynn@twmu.ac.jp.

essential to investigate human osteoclastogenesis using human cells; differences in the species used in studies are critical to discuss the function of cytokines. We, therefore, coined the novel term 'human osteoclastology' to describe studies on human osteoclastogenesis. In this chapter, we focus on the pathogenic roles of Th17 cells in osteoclastogenesis and RA.

Keywords: IL-17, Th17, osteoclast, arthritis, osteoclastogenesis

INTRODUCTION

Rheumatoid arthritis (RA) is a chronic inflammatory disease characterized by synovitis and the destruction of both articular cartilage and bone [1, 2]. Monocyte/macrophage-derived cytokines, including tumor necrosis factor-alpha (TNF-α), interleukin-1 (IL-1), and IL-6, and T-cell-derived cytokine, IL-17, are involved in the induction of osteoclasts and synovitis in RA. Cytokine-mediated osteoclastogenesis and inflammation occur in the joints and synovial tissue [3, 4].

IL-17 is considered a pro-inflammatory cytokine that contributes to the pathogenesis of many autoimmune and inflammatory diseases such as RA [5, 6, 7]. The IL-17 cytokines are collected in a family composed of six members: IL-17A to IL-17F. IL-17A acts locally on osteoclasts and synoviocytes, contributing to bone destruction and synovitis [8, 9].

In the study of human disease, it is essential to investigate human osteoclastogenesis using human cells; differences in the species used in studies are critical to discuss the function of cytokines. We, therefore, coined the novel term 'human osteoclastology' to describe studies on human osteoclastogenesis [10].

In this chapter, we focus on the pathogenic roles of Th17 cells in osteoclastogenesis and RA.

IL-17 IN RA

In 1999, we first reported that IL-17 induces osteoclastogenesis from monocytes through the expression of the NF-κB ligand (RANKL) on osteoblasts using mouse cells [6]. The expression of RANKL is induced by prostaglandin E2 (PGE2) in osteoblasts mediated by IL-17, which is inhibited by NS398, a selective COX-2 inhibitor. Thus, IL-17 indirectly induces osteoclastogenesis via osteoblasts in this manner [6]. We have also reported that the concentration of IL-17 in synovial fluid is significantly increased in RA patients compared with osteoarthritis (OA), trauma, and gout patients [6]. It was also reported that expressions of IL-17 mRNA and protein are higher in RA joints than in healthy controls [11, 12].

Other studies found a high expression of IL-17R in synovial endothelial cells in RA patients [13, 14]. IL-17 directly induces the differentiation of osteoclasts from monocytes and up-regulates RANKL synthesis by RA fibroblast-like synoviocytes (FLS) [15]. IL-17 plays an important role in joint destruction in animal models [16], and IL-17-producing T cells (Th17) also play a crucial role in bone destruction [5]. Th17 cytokine promoted bone erosion in collagen arthritis in murine synovia and bone marrow. IL-17 increased the RANKL/osteoprotegerin (OPG) ratio by stimulating RANKL. We reported that activated T cells expressing RANKL induced osteoclastogenesis [17] and IL-17 directly induced human osteoclast differentiation from human monocytes alone, via TNF-α or the RANK-RANKL pathway [19].

IL-17-induced osteoclastogenesis was inhibited not only by OPG but also by anti-TNF-α antibody [18]. TNF-α, as well as RANKL, was involved in the osteoclastogenesis. IL-17 promotes the expression of RANK on synoviocytes and osteoblasts and activates RANK signaling in osteoclasts [19-21]. Uluckan O et al. found that IL-17A could inhibit osteoblasts and synoviocytes and activate RANK signaling in osteoclasts [22].

IL-17 contributes to the process of angiogenesis by stimulating FLS to produce vascular endothelial growth factor (VEGF) in the presence of RA [23]. IL-17 induced IL-6, IL-8, granulocyte colony-stimulating factor (G-

CSF), and PGE2 from FLS [24]. IL-17 increased the secretion of IL-1β, IL-6, and TNF-α by human macrophages upon stimulation with recombinant protein and increased production of matrix metalloproteinase (MMP)-1, 2, 9 and 13 in synovia, FLS, and cartilage [12, 25].

Chabaud M et al. reported that IL-17 triggers the production of IL-6 by RA synovia, and the addition of an anti-IL-17 antibody to RA synovia cultures decreases MMP-1 production and collagenase activity, suggesting the direct contribution of IL-17 to bone destruction [25]. Moreover, they showed that IL-17 promotes cartilage destruction at the expense of cartilage synthesis [26]. IL-17 alone, or with IL-1 or TNF-α, increases the production of IL-6 by RA bone explants [26, 27]. IL-17 induces synoviocyte activation with increased IL-6 and IL-8, and IL-17 triggers synoviocyte migration and promotes cartilage matrix destruction and bone erosion [8, 28, 29]. Kochi et al. showed that CCR6, a surface marker of Th17 cells at 6q27, is associated with RA susceptibility [30]. Th17 cells express both CCR6 and CCR20, and CCR 20 is also expressed in FLS from RA patients [31]. Monocytes expressing both RANK and CCR6 play an important role in bone destruction of RA [4].

Macrophage inflammatory protein-3 α (MIP-3 α /CCL20) has been reported to preferentially attract Th17 cells (via CCR6 binding) to inflamed rheumatoid joints [31]. It was reported that the RANKL concentration was elevated in RA bone marrow (BM) plasma in comparison with OA BM plasma [15]. The increased production of IL-17A in RA BM may be associated with bone and cartilage destruction in RA [32].

THE SYNERGISTIC EFFECT OF IL-17 AND OTHER CYTOKINES

TNF-α release from monocytes stimulated by IL-17 markedly contributed to IL-17-induced osteoclastogenesis. We reported the synergistic effect of both TNF-α and RANKL on osteoclastogenesis in RA [18]. We demonstrated a synergistic effect on "human" osteoclastogenesis in cultures of CD11b-positive cells. The presence of both sRANKL and TNF-α markedly enhanced osteoclastogenesis, even when the level of either cytokine was low [18].

Fischer JA et al. found that IL-17 and TNF-α have synergistic effects in promoting the production of IL-6, IL-8, granulocyte-colony stimulating factor (G-CSF), and MMPs [33]. TNF-α potentiates the effect of IL-17 on IL-6 and IL-8-induced secretion by rheumatoid synoviocytes [20]. The combination of TNF-α and IL-17 induced GM-CSF secretion by FLS, although TNF- α alone or IL-17 alone showed no effect on GM-CSF secretion [34]. Koenders et al. using mouse models, reported that the combination of a soluble IL-17 receptor and TNF-binding protein inhibited joint destruction more markedly than either of the two anti-cytokine treatments alone [35]. In in vitro study, IL-1β and IL-17 showed synergistic effects on the production of IL-6 by synoviocytes from RA. In addition, IL-1β and IL-17 synergistically induce chemokine (C-C motif) ligand-20 production, which recruits Th17 cells [36]. In mouse models, overexpression of IL-17 and TNF- α caused the dysregulation of IL-1β and MMP mRNA and aggravated joint inflammation [35]. In collagen-induced arthritis mouse models, blocking of IL-17A and IL-1β reduced joint inflammation, bone destruction, and synovitis, which demonstrated the synergistic effect of IL-17 and IL-1β on RA bone destruction [37, 38]. Chabaud and Miossec reported that the blockade of TNF- α combined with the blockade of both IL-17 and IL-1 is more effective in preventing bone destruction ex vivo, indicating that IL-17, TNF- α, and IL-1 have independent effects on osteoclasts [39].

IL-17 INHIBITION

Raza et al. [40] found that early RA of a 3-month duration or less (mean: 9 weeks) is characterized by a distinct and transient synovial fluid cytokine profile of T cells, including IL-17 but not IFN-γ. This indicates that the disease duration of RA is important for the role of cytokines in inflammation and bone destruction. Kokkonen et al. showed that the serum concentration of IL-17 in individuals 3.3 years before onset was significantly higher than in patients 7.7 months after RA onset [41]. Rosu et al. [42] reported that IL-17A levels in synovial fluid are higher than serum levels in early RA patients. In addition, IL-17 and its receptor are up-regulated within ectopic lymphoid in synovia, and these structures play an important role in local inflammation and erosion. Patients were showing no response to TNF-α inhibitors had high circulating Th17 cell numbers [43-45]. IL-17 inhibition showed a high degree of heterogeneity in RA patients; thus, IL-17 inhibition may not be effective for patients with low expression of IL-17. Taken together, IL-17 inhibition may be sufficient in the pre-onset or early stage of RA.

TH17/TREG BALANCE

In RA, the Th17/Treg axis imbalance also plays an important role in the pathogenesis.

Vasilev et al., in an in vitro study, reported that adipose tissue mesenchymal stem cell (AT-MSC) secretory factors down-regulated Th17 and increased Treg cells in peripheral blood mononuclear cells (PBMC) from RA patients [46]. Maseda et al. demonstrated that PGE2 with TGF-β induced Th17 polarization into Tregs [47]. Komatsu et al. reported that IL-17-expressing Treg cells, a product of CD4+Foxp3+ conversion into Th17, exert marked effects on bone destruction [7]. Th17 and Treg exhibit plasticity [48, 49].

THE PLASTICITY OF TH17 CELLS IN THE PATHOGENESIS OF RA

Th17 cells differentiate into Th1 cells (i.e., "non-classic Th1 cells"), and these are more pathogenic than Th17 cells per se. Maggi et al. found that Th17 cells, which express TNFα, can shift to non-classic Th1 cells in an autocrine or a paracrine manner [50]. Chalan et al. demonstrated that the numbers of circulating CD4+CD161+T lymphocytes are elevated in seropositive arthralgia before the onset of RA; on the other hand, they decreased in patients with newly diagnosed RA [51]. In 2016, using peripheral blood from untreated and early-onset RA patients, we demonstrated that the ratio of CD161+Th1 cells (Th17-derived Th1 cells) (Figure 1) to CD161+Th17 cells was elevated [52].

We also reported that the ratio of IFNγ+Th17 cells (Figure 2) in memory Th cells was inversely correlated with the levels of anti-CCP antibodies in untreated and early-onset RA patients [53]. We also evaluated CD161 as a marker of human Th17 cells by measuring the expression of CD161 in human Th17 cells [53]. In addition, we found the detection of IFNγ+IL-17+cells in salivary glands of patients with Mikulicz's disease and Sjogren's syndrome [54]. The plasticity of Th17 cells should be considered not only in RA but also in other autoimmune diseases. Anti-IL-17 antibodies should be used in early-phase RA patients because Th17 cells shift to pathogenic Th17/Th1 or nonclassic Th1, even in the early phase of RA [48, 52, 53, 55]. Thus, target therapy and pharmaceutical development should consider this plasticity.

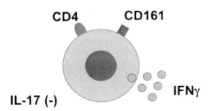

Figure 1. CD161+Th1 (Th17-derived Th1, non-classic Th1 cells).

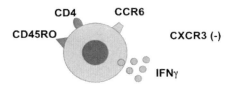

Figure 2. IFNγ+Th17 cells.

THE INHIBITION OF TH17 DIFFERENTIATION

The IL-6 pathway is important in Th17 differentiation, and anti-IL-6 therapy leads to reduced Th17 cells [56]. The JAK/STAT pathway is also important in Th17 differentiation [57]. In vitro, CD4+ T cells incubated with tofacitinib showed inhibited differentiation into Th17 cells. RORγt is a transcription factor required to induce IL-17 transcription by Th17 cells. In murine and human CD4+ T cells and also in murine models, RORγt inhibitor inhibited Th17 differentiation [58, 59]. An IL-1 receptor antagonist and methotrexate (MTX) also decreased levels of Th17 in patients with RA [60]. The anti-CD20 antibody Rituximab decreased Th 17 cells in RA patients [61].

ANTI-IL-17 THERAPY IN RA

Wei et al. reported in a meta-analysis that the IL-17-blocking antibody is effective for ameliorating RA symptoms and reducing ACR20 and ACR 50 (51). Kunwer et al. also reported a systemic review and meta-analysis on the safety and efficacy of anti-IL-17 agents in RA [62]. The meta-analysis of ACR 20 and ACR 50 showed significant heterogeneity [62]. RTC showed the effectiveness of anti-17 for RA patients [63]. Secukinumab reduced disease activity in RA patients who showed an inadequate response to TNF inhibitors in a phase III study [64, 65]. On the other hand, Dokoupilova et al. found that Secukinumab did not provide a benefit to active RA patients who showed an inadequate response to TNF inhibitors in phase III study [66].

In 2017, Lee et al. reported associations between circulating IL-17 levels and RA and between IL-17 gene polymorphism and disease susceptibility based on a meta-analysis [67].

IL-23 IN RA

IL-23 exists upstream of IL-17. We showed that IL-17 production, but not IFN-γ, is dose-dependently induced from human activated T cells stimulated with IL-23 [68] and anti-IL-17 antibody, OPG, and a TNF-α inhibitor blocked IL-23-induced osteoclast differentiation [68]. The inductive effect of IL-17 and the inhibitory effect of IFN-γ on osteoclastogenesis indicated that the balance of these cytokines is important [68]. This balance may be critical in IL-17 and IL-23-induced osteoclastogenesis [68, 69]. We demonstrated that IL-23 directly induces human osteoclastogenesis in the absence of exogenous sRANKL of osteoblasts, that anti-IL-23 antibody administered at a later stage significantly reduces the paw volume dose-dependently in CIA rats, and that anti-IL-23 antibody reduces synovitis and bone destruction in CIA rats [68]. Thus, IL-23 inhibitor may be effective in attenuating synovial inflammation and joint destruction even after the onset of RA [68]. Kim et al. reported that IL-23p19 levels in synovial fluid and sera are higher in RA patients than OA patients and that IL-17 stimulates IL-23p19 mRNA and protein expression in FLS in RA [70]. Lie et al. found that TNF-α and IL-1β stimulated the production of IL-23p19 from RA FLS [71]. Moreover, Il-17 and TNF-α synergistically induce IL-23p19 mRNA expression in FLS [72]. Zaky et al. showed that IL-23 levels of sera are elevated in erosive RA patients and the IL-23p19 concentration correlates with that of IL-17 in sera and synovial fluid [73]. Anti-IL-17 and anti-IL-23 antibodies have marked effectiveness for AS and PsA. The IL-23 inhibitor guselkumab, a human IgG1 antibody against the p19 subunit of IL-23, did not lead to significant improvement in RA [74]. IL-23 may be effective only at the onset of arthritis in RA.

CONCLUSION

It is clear that Th17 cells play a crucial role in the pathogenesis of osteoclastogenesis and RA. The results of anti-IL-17 therapy showed significant heterogeneity in RA patients. The plasticity of Th17 plays an important role in the pathogenesis of RA. It is necessary to select RA patients who have highly bioactive IL-17 to obtain a sufficient effect of the anti-IL-17 antibody. IL-17 inhibition may be sufficient in the pre-onset or early stage of RA. Clarifying these issues will help develop strategies for a novel therapeutic approach.

REFERENCES

[1] Nanke Y, Kotake S, Akama H, Kamatani N Alkaline phosphatase in rheumatoid arthritis patients: possible contribution of bone-type ALP to the rased activities of ALP in rheumatoid arthritis patients. *Clin Rheumaol* 2002;21(3):198-202.

[2] Nanke Y, Kobashigawa T, Yago T, Kawamot M, Yamanaka H, Kotake S. A novel peptide from TCTA protein inhibits proliferation of fibroblast-like synoviocyte (FLS) from rheumatoid arthritis patients. *Cent Eur J Immunol* 2014;39:468-470.

[3] Nanke Y, Kobashigawa T, Yago T, Kawamoto M, Yamanaka H, Kotake S. Tumor necrosis factor a and matrix metalloproteinase-3 production in rheumatoid arthritis synovial tissue is inhibited by clocking gap junction communication. *Cent Eur J Immuno.* 2012;37(3):237-242.

[4] Nanke Y, Kobahigawa T, Yago T, Kawamoto M, Yamanaka H, Kotake S. RANK expression and osteoclstogenesis in human monocytes in peripheral bold form rheumatoid arthritis patients. *Biomed Res Int.* 2016;2016:4874195.

[5] Sato K, Suematsu A, Okamot K, Yamaguchi A, Morishita Y, Kadono Y et al. Th17 function as an osteoclastogenic helper T cell subset

that links T cell activation and bone destruction. *J Exp Med* 2006;203:2673-2682.

[6] Kotake S, Udagawa N, Takahashi N, Matsuzaki K, Itoh K, Isiyama S et al. IL-17 in synovial fluids from patients with rheumatoid arthritis is a potent stimulator of osteoclastogenesis. *J Clin Invest* 1999.103;1345-52.

[7] Komatsu N, Okamoto K, Sawa S et al. Pathogenic conversion of Foxp3+T cells into Th17 cells in autoimmune arthritis. *Nat Med* 2014; 20:62-68.

[8] Hot A, Zrioual S, Toh ML, Leniel V, Miossec P. Il-17A-versus Il-17F in cued intracellular signal transduction pathways and modulation by IL-17RA and IL-17RC RNA interference in rheumatoid synoviocytes. *Ann Rheum Dis.* 2011; 70:341-8.

[9] Ndongo-Thiam N, Miossec P. A cell-based bioassay for circulating bioactive Il-17:application to destruction in rheumatoid arhtirits. *Ann Rheum Dis.* 2015;74:1629-31.

[10] Kotake S, Nanke Y, Yago T, Kawamoto M, Yamanaka H. Human osteoclastogenic T cells and human osteoclastology (Editorial). *Arthritis Rheum.* 2009; 60:3158-3163.

[11] Shahrara S, Huang Q, Mandelin AM, Pope RM. TH-17 cells in rheumatoid arthritis. *Arthritis Reseach & ther.* 2008; 10(4): R93.

[12] Moran EM, Mullan R, McCormick J, Connolly Ml Sullivan O, Fitzgerald O et al. Human rheumatoid arthritis tissue production of IL-17 A drives matrix and cartilage degradation: synergy with fumor necrosis factor-alpha, oncostatin M and response to biologic therapies. *Arthritis Res Ther* 2009; 11:R113.doi: 10.1186/ar2772.

[13] Chabaud M, Durand JM, Buchs N, Fossiez F, Page G, Frappart L et al. Human interleukin17: A T cell-derived proinflammatory cytokine produced by the rheumatoid arthritis synovium. *Arthritis Rheum* 1999.42:963-70.

[14] Honorati MC, Meliconi R, pulsaelli L, Cane S, Frizziero L, FacchiniA. High in vivo expression of interleukin-17 receptor in synovial endothelial cells and chondrocytes from arthritis patients. *Rheumatology* 2001; 40;422-7.

[15] Kim KW, Kim HR, Kim BM, Cho ML, Lee SH. Th17 cytokine regulates osteoclastogenesis in rheumatoid arthritis. *Am J Pathol* 2015; 185(11): 3011-24.

[16] Lubberts E, Koenders MI, van den Berg WB. The role of T cell interleukin-17 in conducting destructive arthritis: lessons from animal models. *Arthritis Res Ther* 2005:7:29-37.

[17] Kotake S, Udagawa N, Hakota M, Mogi M, Yano K, Tsuda E et al. Activated human T cells directly induce osteoclasogenesis from human monocytes: possible role of T cells in bone destruction in rheumatoid arthritis patients. *Arthritis Rheuma* 2001; 44:1003-1012.

[18] Yago, T, Nanke Y, Ichikawa N, Kobashigawa T, Mogi M, Kamatani N et al. IL-17 induces osteoclastogenesis from human monocytes alone in the absence of osteoblasts, which is potently inhibited by anti-TNF-alpha antibody: A novel mechanism of osteoclastogenesis by IL-17. *J Cell Biochem* 2009: 108:947-955.

[19] Van Bezooijen RL, Papapouos SE, Lowik CW. Effect of interleukin-17 on nitric oxide production and osteoclastic bone resorption: is there dependency on nuclear factor-kappaB and receptor activator of nuclear factor kappaB (RANK/RANK signaling? *Bone* 2001; 28:378-86.

[20] Lovocat F, Maggi L, Annunziato F, Miossec P. T-cell clones from Th1, Th17 or Th1/Th17 lineages and their signature cytokines have different capacity to activate endothelial cells or synoviocytes. *Cytokine* 2016; 88:241-50.

[21] Lovacat F, Osta B, Miossec P. Increased sensitivity of rheumatoid synoviocytes to Schnurri-3 expression in TNF-alpha and IL-17A induced osteoblastic differentiation. *Bone.* 2016; 87:89-96.

[22] Uluckan O, Jimenez M, Karbach S, Jeschke A, Grana O, Keller J et al. Chronic skin inflammation leads to bone loss by IL-17-mediated inhibition of Wnt signaling in osteoblasts. *Sci Transl Med.* 2016; 8:330ra37.

[23] Ryu S, Lee JH, Kim SL. IL-17 increased the production of vascular endothelial growth factor in rheumatoid arthritis synoviocytes. *Clin Rheumaol* 2005; 25(1):16-20.

[24] Fossiez F, Djossou O, Chomarat P, Flores-Romo L, Ait-Yahia S, Maat C et al. T cell interleukin-17 induces stromal cells to produce proinflammatory and hematopoietic cytokine. *J Exp Med* 1996; 183(6):2593-603.

[25] Chabaud M, Garnero P, Dayer JM, Guerne PA, Fossiez F, Miossec P et al. Contribution of interleukin 17 to synovium matrix destruction in rheumatoid arthritis. *Cytokine* 2000; 12:1092-9.

[26] Chabaud M, Lubberts E, Joosten L, van Den Berg W, Miossec P. IL-17 derived from juxta-articular bone and synovium contributes to joint degradation in rheumatoid arthritis. *Arthritis Res* 2001; 3:168-77.

[27] Osta B, Roux JP, Lavocat F, Pierre M, Ndongo-Thim N, Boivin G et al. Differential effects of IL-17A and INF-alpha on osteoblastic differentiation of isolated synoviocytes and on bone explants from arthritis patients. *Front Immunol* 2015; 6:151. Doi: 10.3389.

[28] Hwang SY, Kim JY, Kim KW, Park MK, Moon Y, Kim WU et al. IL-17 induces production of IL-6 and Il-8 in rheumatoid arthritis synovial fibroblasts via NF-kappaB- and PI3-kinase/Akt-dependent pathways. *Arthritis Res Ther* 2004; 6:R120-8.

[29] Zrioual S, Toh ML, Touranadre A, Zhou Y, Cazalis MA, Pachot A et al. IL-17RA and IL-17RC receptors are essential for IL-17A-induced ELR+CXC chemokine expression in syoviocytes and are overexpressed in rheumatoid blood. *J Immunol* 2008; 180:655-63.

[30] Kochi Y, Okada Y, Suzuki A. A regulatory variant in CCR6 is associated with rheumatoid arthritis susceptibility. *Nature Geneticis.* 2010;42(6):515-520.

[31] Hirota K, Yoshitomi H, Hashimoto M, Naeda S, Teradaira S, Sugimoto N et al. Preferential recruitment of CCR6-expressing Th17 cells to inflamed joints via CCL20 in rheumatoid arthritis and its animal model. *J Exp Med* 2007; 204(12):2803-12.

[32] Kuca-Warnawin E, Kurowska W, Prochorec-Sobieszek M, Radzikowska A, Burakowski T et al. Rheumatoid arthritis bone marrow environment supports Th17 response. *Arthritis Reseach & Ther* 2017; 19:274.

[33] Lee YH, Bae SC. Associations between circulating IL-17 levels and rheumatoid arthritis and between IL-17 gene polymorphisms and disease susceptibility: A meta-analysis. *Postgrad. Med J* 2017.

[34] Fossiez F,Djossou O, Chomarat P, Flores-Romas L, Ait-Yahia S, Maat C et al. T cell interleukin-17 induces stromal cells to produce proinflmmatory and hematopoietic cytokines. *J Exp Med* 1996;183(6):2593-603.

[35] Koenders MI, Marijnissen RJ, Joosten LAB, Abdollahi-Roodsaz S, Di Padova FE, van de Loos FA et al. T cell lessons form the rheumatoid arthritis synovium SCID mouse model. *Arthritis Rheum* 2012; 64(6):1762-70.

[36] Chabaud M, Page G, Miossec P. Enhancing effect of IL-1, IL-17, and TNF-alpha on macrophage inflammatory protein-3alpha production in rheumatoid arthritis: regulation by soluble receptors and Th 2 cytokines. *J Immunol* 2001:167:6015-20.

[37] Zhang Y, Ren G, Guo M, Ye X, Zhao J, Xu L et al. Synergistic effects of interleukin-beta and interleukin-17A antibodies on collagen-induced arthritis mouse model. *Int Immunoopharmacol.* 2013; 15:199-205.

[38] Wu Q, Wang Y, Wang Q, Yu D, Wang Y, Song L et al. The bispecific antibody aims at the vicious circle of IL-1 beta and IL-17A, is beneficial for the collagen-induced rheumatoid arthritis of mice through NF-kappaB signaling pathway. *Immunol Lett.* 2016; 179:68-79.

[39] Chabaud M, Miossec P. The combination of tumor necrosis factor alpha blockade with interleukin-1 and interleukin-17 blockade is most effective for controlling synovial inflammation and bone resorption in an ex vivo model. *Arthrits Rheum* 2001; 44:1293-1303.

[40] Rasa K, Falciani F, Curnow SJ, Ross EJ, Lee CY, Akbar AN et al. Early rheumatoid arthritis is characterized by a distinct and transient synovial fluid cytokine profile of T cell and stromal cell origin. *Arthritis res Ther* 2005;7:R784-795.

[41] Kokkonen H, Soderstrom I, Rocklov J, Hallmans G, Lejon K, Rantapaa Dahlqvist S et al. Up-regulation of cytokines and

chemokines predates the onset of rheumatoid arthritis. *Arthritis Rheum* 2010; 62:383-391.

[42] Rosu A, Margaritescu C, Stepan A, MusetescuA, Ene M. IL-17 patterns in synovium, serum and synovial fluid from treatment-native, early rheumatoid arthritis patients. *Rom J Morphol Embryol.* 2012; 53:73-80.

[43] Aerts NE, de Knop KJ, Leysen J, Ebo DG, Bridts CH, Weyler JJ et al. Increased IL-17 production by peripheral T helper cells after tumor necrosis factor blockade in rheumatoid arthritis is accompanied by inhibition of migration-associated chemokine receptor expression. *Rheumaotology.* 2010; 49(12):2264-72.

[44] Chen DY, Chen YM, Chen HH, Hsieh CW, Lin CC, Lan JL. Increasing levels of circulating Th17 cells and interleukin-17 in rheumatoid arthritis patients with an inadequate response to anti-TNF-α therapy. *Arthritis Rheum* 2011;63(10): 2939-48.

[45] Alzabin S, Abraham SM, Taher TE, Paflreeman A, Hull D, MaName K et al. Incomplete response of inflammatory arthritis to TNF-a blockade is associated with the Th17 pathway. *Ann Rheum Dis* 2012; 64(8):2499-503.

[46] Vasilev G, Ivanova M, Ivanova-Todorova E, Tumangelova-Yuzeir K, Krasimirova E, Stoilov R et al. Secretory factors produced by adipose mesenchmal stem cells down regulate Th17 and increase Treg cells in peripheral blood mononuclear cells from rheumatoid arthritis patients. *Rheumatol Int* 2019 https://doi.org/10.1007.

[47] Maseda D, Banerjee A, Johnson EM, Washington MK, Kim H, Lau KS et al. mPGE-1-mediated production of PGE2 and EP4 receptor sensing regulate T cell colonic inflammation. *Front Immunol* 2018; 9:2954.

[48] Malemud CJ. Defective T-cell apoptosis and T-regulatory cell dysfunction in rheumatoid arthritis. *Cells.* 2018; 7:223.

[49] Fontenot JD, Rasmussen JP, Williams LM, Dooley JL, Farr AG, Rudensky AY. Regulatory T cell lineage specification by the forehead transcription factor Foxp3. *Immunity* 2005; 22:329-341.

[50] Wei M, Duan D. Effecacy and safety of monoclonal antibodies targeting interleukin-17 pathway for inflammatory arthritis: a meta-analysis of randomized controlled clinical trails. *Drug Design, Develop Ther* 2016;10:2771-2777.

[51] Chalan P, Kroesen BJ, van der Geest KS, Huitema MG, Abdulahad WH, Bijzet J et al. Circulating CD4+CD161+ T lymphocytes are increased in seropositive arthralgia patients but decrease in patients with newly diagnosed rheumatoid arhtirits. *Plos ONE* 2013;8:e79370.

[52] Kotake S, Nanke Y, Yago T, Kawamoto M, Kobashigawa T, Yamanaka H. Elevated ratio of Th17 cell-derived Th1 cells (CD161+Th1 cells) to CD161+Th17 cells in peripheral blood of early-onset rheumatoid arhtiritis. *Bio Med Inter* 2016;2016:4186027.

[53] Kotake S, Yago T, Kobashigawa T, Nanke Y. The plasticity of Th17 cells in the pathogenesis of rheumatoid arhtirits. *J Clin. Med* 2017;10:6(7).

[54] Nanke Y, Kobashigawa T, Yago T, Kawamoto M, Yamanaka H, Kotake S. Detection of IFN-g+IL-17+ cells in salivary glands of patients with sjogren's syndrome and MikulicZ's disease. Potential role of Th17Th1 in the pathogenesis of autoimmune disease *Nihon Rinsho Meneki Gakki Kaishi* 2016;36:473-477.

[55] Kotake S, Nanke Y, Yago T, Kawamot M, Kobashigawa T, Yamanaka H. Ratio of circulating IFNγ+ "Th17 cells" in memory Th cells is inversely correlated with the titer of anti-CCP antibodies in early-onset rheumatoid arthritis patients base on flow cytometry methods of the human immunology project. *Bio Med Research Inter* 2016;2016:9694289.

[56] Samson M, Audia S, Janikashvili N, Ciudad M, Trad M, Fraszczak J et al. Inhibition of interleukin-6 function corrects Th17/Treg cell imbalance in patients with rheumatoid arthritis. *Arthritis Rheum* 2012; 64(8):2499-503.

[57] Maesima K, Uamaoka K, Kubo S, Nakano K, Iwata S, Saito K et al. The JAK inhibitor Tofacitinib regulates synovitis through inhibition

of interferon-γ and interleukin -17 productions by human CD4+ T cells. *Arthritis Rheum* 2012;64(6):1790-8.

[58] Fugita-Sato S, Ito S, Isobe T, Ohyama T, Wakabayashi K, Morishita K et al. Structural basis of digoxin that antagonizes ROR t receptor activity and suppresses Th17 cell differentiation and interleukin (IL)-17 production. *J Biol Chem* 2011; 286:31409-17.

[59] Huh JR, Leung MW, Huang P, Ryan DA, Krout MR, Malapaka RR et al. Digoxin and its derivatives suppress Th17 cell differentiation by antagonizing RORγt activity. *Nature* 2011; 472(7344):486-90.

[60] Niu X, He D, Deng S, Li W, Xi Y, Xie C et al. Regulatory immune responses induced by IL-1 receptor antagonist in rheumatoid arthritis. *Mol Immunol* 2011; 49(1-2): 290-6.

[61] Van de Veerdong FL, Lauwaerys B, Marijnissen RJ, Timmermans K, Di Padova F, koenders MI et al. The anti-CD20 antibody Rituximab reduces the Th17 cell response. *Arthritis Rheum* 2011; 63(6): 1507-16.

[62] Kunwar S, Dahal K, Sharma S. Anti-IL-17 therapy in treatment of rheumatoid arthritis: a systemic literature review and meta-analysis of randomized controlled trial. *Rheumatol Int* 2016; 36:1065-1075.

[63] Genovese MC, Green Wald M, Cho C-S et al. Phase II randomized study of subcutaneous ixekizumab, an anti-interleukin-17 monoclonal antibody, in rheumatoid arthritis patients who were naïve to biologic agent or had an inadequate response to tumor necrosis factor inhibitors. *Arthritis Rheumatol Hoboken NJ.* 2014; 66:1693-1704.

[64] Blanco FJ, Moricke R, Dokoupilova E, Codding C, Neal J, Andersson M et al. Secukinumab in active rheumatoid arthritis: A phase III randomized, Double- Blind, active comparator- and Placebo-controlled study. *Arthritis Rheum* 2017; 69(6): 1144-1153.

[65] Tahir H, Deodhar A, Genovese M, Takechi T, Aelion J, Van den Bosch F et al. Secukinumab in active rheumatoid arthritis after anti-TNF α therapy: a randomized, double-blind placebo-controlled phase 3 study. *Rheumatol Ther* 2017; 4(2): 475-488.

[66] Dokoupilova E, Aelion J, Takeuchi T, Malavolta N, Sfikakis PP, Wang Yet al. Secukinumab after anti-tumor necrosis factor-a therapy: a phase III study in active rheumatoid arthritis. *Scand J Rheumaol* 2018; 47(4): 276-281.

[67] Fischer JA, hueber AJ, Wilson S, Galm M, Baum W,Kitson C et al. Combined inhibition of tumor necrosis factor a and interleukin-17 as a therapeutic opportunity in rheumatoid arthritis: Development and characterization of a novel bispecific antibody. *Arhtirits Rheum* 2015;67:51-62.

[68] Yago T, Nanke Y, Kowamoto M, Furuya T, Kobashigawa T, Kamatani N et al. IL-23 induces human osteoclastogenesis via IL-17 in vitro, and anti IL-23 antibody attenuates collagen-induced arthritis in rats. *Arthritis Res Ther* 2007; 99;R96.

[69] Kokake S, Nanke Y, Mogi M, Kawamoto M, Furuya T, Yago T et al. IFN-γ-producing human T cells directly induce osteoclastogenesis from human monocytes via the expression of RANKL. *Eur J Immunol.* 2005;35:3353-3363.

[70] Kim HR, Cho ML, Kim KW, Juhn JY, Hwang SY, Yoon CH et al. Up-regulation of IL-23p19 expression in rheumatoid arthritis synovial fibroblasts by IL-17 through PI3-kinase-, NFkappaB-and p38 MAPK-dependent signaling pathway. *Rheumaology* 2007; 46:57-64.

[71] Liu FL, Chen CH, Chu SJ, Chen JH, Lai JH, Sytwu HK et al. Interleukin-23p19 expression induced by IL-1beta in human fibroblast-like synoviocytes with rheumatoid arthritis via active nuclear factor-kappaB and AP-1 dependent pathway. *Rheumatology* 2007; 46:1266-1273.

[72] Goldberg M, Nadiv O, Luknar-Gabor N, Agar G, Beer Y, Katz Y et al. Synergism between tumor necrosis factor alpha and interleukin-17 to induce Il-23p19 expression in fibroblast-like synoviocytes. *Mol Immunol* 2009; 46:1854-1859.

[73] Zaly DS, EL-Nahrery EM. Role of interleukin-23 as a biomarker in rheumatoid arthritis patients and its correlation with disease activity. *Int Imunopharmacol* 2016; 31:105-108.

[74] Smolen JS, Agarwal SK, Livanova E, Xu XL, Miao Y, Zhuang Y et al. A randomized phase II study evaluation the efficacy and safety of subcutaneously administered ustekinumab and guselkumab in patients with active rheumatoid arthritis despite treatment with methotrexate. *Ann Rheum Dis.* 2017; 76:831-839.

In: Th17 Cells in Health and Disease
Editor: Tsvetelina Velikova

ISBN: 978-1-53617-152-5
© 2020 Nova Science Publishers, Inc.

Chapter 3

PHENOTYPIC AND FUNCTIONAL HETEROGENEITY OF TH17 CELLS IN SYSTEMIC SCLEROSIS

Rositsa V. Karalilova, MD, PhD*

Department of Internal Diseases, Medical University of Plovdiv,
University Hospital "Kaspela",
Clinic of Rheumatology, Plovdiv, Bulgaria

ABSTRACT

Systemic sclerosis (SSc) is an autoimmune disorder of the connective tissue that is characterized by autoantibody production, vasculopathy, and extreme deposition of collagen in the skin and internal organs.

Despite the still unclear pathogenetic complexity of SSc, various new pathways have been investigated in the last years. The role of T lymphocytes with an abnormal immune response in SSc is well established. IL-17- producing helper T (Th17) cell and regulatory T (Treg) cell subsets play determinant roles in SSc pathogenesis. Th17 cell subsets are involved and up-regulate processes such as inflammation,

---

* Corresponding Author's Email: karalilova@hotmail.com.

fibrosis, and autoimmunity. Treg cell subsets, on the other hand, have an immunosuppressive function and inhibit the immunological performance of Th17 cells. Current evidence suggests that the imbalance and abnormal functions of Th17/Treg cells may contribute to SSc. Therefore, this chapter aims to overview the current understanding of the Th17/Treg differentiation and functions and their roles in the SSc pathogenesis.

Keywords: systemic sclerosis, Th17 cells, autoimmunity

INTRODUCTION

Systemic sclerosis (SSc) is an autoimmune disease characterized by inflammation, vascular abnormalities, production of autoantibodies, and extracellular matrix deposition [1]. Excessive uncontrolled collagen deposition results in skin and inner organs fibrosis with alterations in both the innate and adaptive immunities. It is known for its early vascular damage followed by both tissue and systemic fibrosis affecting many organs, including, in particular, the skin, lungs, heart, kidneys, and digestive tract [2]. The combination of environmental factors and genetic background seems to contribute to the development of this disease.

Despite the still unclear pathogenetic complexity of SSc, various new pathways have been investigated in the last years.

The immune system is directly involved in the pathogenesis of SSc. The observations supporting this statement are the presence of autoantibodies (autoAb) directed against auto-antigens in the sera of SSc individuals. Another reason is that clinical features characteristically present in SSc are shared with other autoimmune systemic conditions such as systemic lupus erythematosus (SLE), rheumatoid arthritis (RA), or overlapping syndromes including mixed connective tissue disease and overlaps with myositis. An enormous amount of work has provided evidence indicating that different cells and soluble mediators present abnormalities that correlate with distinct SSc phenotypes. They may be pathologically linked to disease development [3].

Activation of the immune system together with microvascular aberrations and increased extracellular matrix deposition in tissues play fundamental roles in the pathogenesis of SSc. Besides, excessive production of antinuclear antibodies (ANA) is also observed. They are detected in almost 90% of patients is a result of abnormal activation of T and B cells. Microvascular and immunological abnormalities are predominant at an early stage of the disease, whereas inflammation and fibrosis are observed in later stages [4].

As a progressive fibrotic disease, SSc is characterized by excessive deposition of extracellular matrix (ECM) components such as collagen and glycoprotein [5]. However, the clinical picture and course of SSc are highly heterogeneous. Although the pathogenesis of the disease remains unknown, central part of pathogenesis takes vascular damage and inflammation. The latter is associated with activated innate and adaptive immunity. All of these mechanisms are involved in the pathological mechanisms underlying the skin and visceral organ fibrosis, specifically the lungs and gastrointestinal tract. Lung fibrosis is a common clinical manifestation of SSc and remains the leading cause of death in affected patients [5].

PATHOGENESIS

Dysregulation of Innate and Adaptive Immunity in SSc

SSc is characterized by the dysregulation of innate and adaptive immunity and the presence of autoantibodies, which is similar to systemic lupus erythematosus (SLE), rheumatoid arthritis (RA), dermatomyositis, bullous diseases, and other autoimmune diseases [6-8]. In SSc, important autoantibodies are produced against angiotensin II type I receptor (AT1R) and endothelin-1 type A receptor (ETAR), which link the skin fibroblasts production of collagen to angiogenesis modulation [7].

The Role of B Cells

The participation of B cells to the immune response is not exclusively mediated by the production of antibodies but includes key activities such as antigen presentation, cytokine secretion, modulation of T cell, and dendritic cell activation [9]. B cell responses are mainly determined by signaling thresholds through the B cell receptor (BcR) complex and are regulated by specific cell surface and cytoplasmic molecules. Abnormal B cell function and homeostasis have been implicated in the onset and progression of different systemic autoimmune disorders. In SSc patients, lesional skin and lung tissues from subjects with ILD demonstrate prominent B cell infiltration [10, 11]. Gene expression studies have shown significant upregulation of B cell-related genes in affected SSc skin [11]. Analysis of circulating B cell repertoire in SSc has shown expansion of the (CD27-) naïve B cell subset and the concurrent decline of memory B cell and plasma cellular components [12]. However, these memory B cells retain a strong immunoglobulin secretory function and exhibit upregulation of co-stimulatory molecules (CD80 and CD86) and CD95, suggesting a chronic activation state and an increased sensitivity to pro-apoptotic stimuli [13, 14]. Accordingly, the expression of positive response regulators such as CD19 and the associated molecule CD21 (complement receptor type 2) is increased in naïve as well as memory B cells of SSc patients compared to healthy controls [13, 15]. A single nucleotide polymorphism (SNP) in the upstream region of the CD19 gene has been associated with higher expression of this molecule in circulating B cells and susceptibility to SSc [16]. A proliferation-inducing ligand (APRIL) and B-cell activating factor (BAFF) are members of the tumor necrosis factor (TNF) superfamily exerting important homeostatic functions on B cells such as maturation, activation, and survival (anti-apoptotic) [17]. Serum levels of BAFF and APRIL are increased in SSc patients compared to controls and are associated with specific clinical manifestations such as extent of skin involvement (BAFF) and the presence of pulmonary fibrosis (APRIL) [18, 19]. The secretion of APRIL from PBMCs was significantly higher in SSc patients compared to controls and was associated with diffuse skin phenotype, the presence of ILD, and anti-SCL70 positivity among other SSc clinical features [19]. Interestingly, BAFF serum levels are increased in the tight-skin (TSK/+) mouse model of SSc, and blockage of the BAFF/BAFF-receptor interaction can prevent the development of skin fibrosis, inhibit autoantibody generation and increase the production of anti-fibrotic cytokines (i.e., IFNg). All these data indicate that B cell activation and overactivity are important features of the immune response in SSc and that an imbalance of B cell homeostasis and function may contribute to the amplification of the inflammatory as well as the fibrotic process in this disease.

T Cells in SSc Pathogenesis

It is known that T lymphocytes play a critical role in the pathogenesis of innate and adaptive immunity [6]. According to their functions, T lymphocytes can be identified as the cytotoxic T cell (CTL) subset, the helper T(Th) cell subset, and the regulatory T (Treg) cell subset. It has been observed that the cells of the Th cell subset, which express the surface marker CD4, direct the adaptive immune responses. The most common Th cell subsets are Th1 and Th2 cells with discrepant immunological behaviors. Naïve Th cells differentiate into Th1 cells, which are co-stimulated by IL-12 when antigen-presenting cells (APCs) are active. Th1 cells enhance the antigen processing pathways by secreting Interferon-gamma (IFN-γ), which promotes further differentiation of Th1 subsets and suppresses the production of other patterns of cytokines. IL-4 directs the differentiation of naïve Th cells into Th2 cells and promotes the expansion of Th2 cells while suppressing other Th cell subsets. Th2 cells primarily produce cytokines IL-4, IL-10, IL-13, and IL-5 [20, 21]. Similar to other autoimmune diseases, the dysregulation of the immune system consists in SSc were classically considered to be the result of alternating Th1 and Th2 subsets or their imbalance [20, 22-29]. However, new evidence suggests the increasing importance of other T cell subsets, such as Th17 and Treg cells, in SSc and other autoimmune diseases.

Injury-induced initiation of vascular endothelial cells activation is the first and principal event of SSc. When activated, vascular endothelial cells can induce the infiltration of inflammatory cells, such as CD4+ T cells in the perivascular tissue. These cells can produce high levels of inflammatory cytokines, such as interleukin 4 (IL-4) [3, 30]. It is thought that CD4+ T cells are involved in the pathogenesis of SSc [158]. In addition to vasculopathy and fibrosis, autoimmunity features are another hallmark of SSc. In the preclinical very early phase, the pathological changes in skin affected by SSc include perivascular edema and in inflammatory cell infiltration [30]. The typical pathological findings in the advanced stage of SSc are augmented dermal fibrosis, reduced amount of capillaries, and loss of skin adnexa [30]. In the lungs affected by SSc, in inflammatory cell infiltration in the interstitium and alveoli precedes evident pulmonary fibrosis [31]. These observations suggest that the infiltration of CD4+ T cells may lead to generalized tissue fibrosis in SSc.

Th17 cells are a relatively recently described subset of CD4+ T helper cells that secrete IL-17A and IL-17F primarily. Th17 cells and the related pathways are involved in the pathogenesis of many inflammatory and autoimmune disorders, such as rheumatoid arthritis, type 1 diabetes, and Sjögren's syndrome [32]. Some authors claim that the production of IL-17 is significantly enlarged in SSc patients compared with healthy controls [33, 34, 40, 157]. IL-17 directly encourages the production of IL-6 and IL-8 in human dermal fibroblasts [35]. In vitro studies have demonstrated that IL-17 up-regulate the proliferation of fibroblasts and IL-1 production in vascular endothelial cells. All these results support the pivotal role of IL-17 in fibrosis and endothelial inflammation [41, 33, 36].

Interestingly, many cytokines that are considered inflammatory, such as TGF-β, IL-6, and IL-1, are known to be involved in the pathogenesis of SSc. Besides, they promote Th17 differentiation. This strongly supports the skewing of CD4+ T cell immune response toward Th17 in the disease. However, existing evidence shown in human and experimental animal models of SSc have failed to reach a definite conclusion [37-39]. Some investigators show that SSc skin biopsy samples were abundant with IL-17+ cells compared to those of healthy controls. It was also demonstrated that IL-17 reduced the myofibroblast transdifferentiation, suggesting its antifibrotic role during dermal fibrosis in SSc [37]. Another study reported the close relationship between SSc disease activity and the number of Th17 cells [40]. The IL-17 cytokine derived from Th17 cells promoted collagen production and fibroblast growth [40]. Contrary to all the above, some studies have not detected differences in IL-17 levels between SSc patients and healthy controls [42, 43].

The IL-17 Cytokine Family

The IL-17 cytokine family consists of six structurally related molecules: IL-17A, IL-17B, IL-17C, IL-17D, IL-17E (IL-25), and IL-17F [44]. IL-17A and IL-17F are produced primarily by immune cells (i.e., T helper cells). The other members: IL-17B, IL-17C, IL-17D, and IL-17E, are mainly provided by a non-T cell source [45]. IL-17A is secreted as a dimer, either IL-17A-IL-17A homodimer or IL-17A-IL-17F heterodimer. IL-17A and IL-17F share more than 50% similarities within structure, although they bind with different affinity to IL-17 receptors on their target cells [46]. As shown above, Th17-derived IL-17 is believed to add to processes such as fibroblast proliferation, production of collagen and recruitment of inflammatory cells to vascular endothelium [36, 47, 48].

Th17 cells, whose differentiation is promoted mainly by IL-6, are characterized by the secretion of the hallmark pro-inflammatory cytokine IL-17 [49, 50]. Induced by different cytokines, there are two functionally distinct Th17 populations: one is the Th17 effector (Teff17) cell, and the other is Th17 regulatory (Treg17) cell [6]. Teff17 cells show pathogenic effects and secrete granulocyte-macrophage colony-stimulating factor (GM-CSF) and IL-22. Treg17 cells seem to be regulatory and protective, producing IL-10 and IL-21, and their development is regulated by the signal transducer and activator of transcription (STAT) 3 [51-54]. Therefore, IL-17 is a group of cytokines with multiple functions, including inflammatory production and tissue-damaging molecules. The role of Th17 cells in mediating tissue inflammation and autoimmunity is prominent because they have a pleiotropic effect on fibroblasts, keratinocytes, endothelial cells, neutrophils, and memory T cells [55].

Recently, Th17 cells and their production cytokines, such as IL-17, IL-21, and IL-22, have been of great interest for their presence and role in SSc. Several groups of researchers observed that the level of Th17 cells and their products in peripheral blood or skin from SSc patients is increased in varying degrees compared with healthy donors [23, 28, 33, 34, 40, 43, 61-67]. Some studies have claimed that the level of Th17 cell subsets is related to disease activity and collagen overproduction and contributes to lung impairment in both mouse models and clinical SSc cases [23, 40, 43, 68].

IL-17A has multiple extensive impacts [20]. It has been reported that IL-17A extracted from SSc patients seems to induce proliferation, synthesis, and the migration of dermal vascular smooth muscle cells (DVSMCs) via the extracellular signal-regulated protein kinases (ERK) signaling pathway [36, 69]. In addition, IL-17A affects three kinds of pro-inflammatory chemokines, which are monocyte chemotactic protein (MCP)-1, IL-8, and matrix metalloproteinases (MMP)-1 [70]. Interestingly, IL-17A seems to increase mainly in SSc skin with low expression in localized scleroderma [65].

It has been recently demonstrated that IL-17A/Th17 cells might play contradictory roles in fibrosis [64, 66, 37, 38, 70-75]. In the context of SSc, some studies claimed that IL-17A/Th17 cells induced the synthesis and secretion of type I collagen to promote the fibrosis of murine SSc skin and lungs, and IL-17A-deficient mice exhibited a protective effect [38, 66]. However, other researchers discovered that in healthy individuals and SSc patients, IL-17A/Th17 cells decreased type I collagen production by dermal fibroblasts as well as the differentiation of fibroblasts into myofibroblasts; they declared the increased Th17 cell counts might be considered not mechanistically linked to fibrosis but by autoimmunity [37, 64, 70]. However, it is still unclear why IL-17A/Th17 cells behave so contrary in a different circumstance. Although IL-17 A/Th17 cells may show anti-fibrotic effects to a certain extent, they seem to fail to counteract the pro-fibrotic mechanisms mediated by other cells and substances, resulting in the fibrotic manifestation in SSc.

Besides the IL-17 family, other members of Th17-derived cytokines also show noticeable associations to SSc. IL-22 is a key pro-inflammatory cytokine in the skin produced by a large amount of Th cells—including Th17—due to its enhancement of killing bacteria and producing cytokines (TNF, IL-1, and IL-12) and chemokines (IL-8 and MCP-1) [20, 76]. IL-21 correlates with the severity of early SSc skin lesions [63]. Some research has proven that the levels of circulating IL-17 and IL-23 are increased in SSc patients [33, 40, 61]. Another group has found that serum IL-23, in addition to IL-17, is decreased while IL-21 is elevated [43]. In any case, there is no doubt that these Th17-derived cytokines play a crucial role in SSc.

Moreover, it has been reported that the gene polymorphisms of CCR6, a surface marker of Th17 cell subsets, are associated with the susceptibility to SSc [77]. All of the above results affirm the pivotal role of Th17 cells and their roles in promoting targeted organ damage in both early and long-standing stages of SSc by contributing to inflammation, fibrosis, and autoimmunity. We can summarize that Th17 cell subsets play mainly a promoting role during the pathogenesis of SSc.

Some researchers discovered that IL-33-matured dendritic cells have more IL-1β and IL-6 secretion, which are involved in Th17 cell differentiation [78]. TLR7 signaling has been found down-regulating Th17 cell differentiation from naive T cells and IL-17 production [79]. IκB kinase (IKK) α-dependent phosphorylation of S376 stimulated retinoic acid-related orphan receptor (ROR) γt function in Th17 differentiation while IKKα-independent phosphorylation of S484 shows inhibition [80]. These recent studies expose that impacts on cytokines, signaling pathways, or protein phosphorylations could participate in the differentiation, proliferation, and function of SSc Th17 cells.

A number of environmental factors are involved in altering Th17 cell responses from protective immunity to promoting inflammation and autoimmune diseases. Responses to bacterial infections in the gut and, potentially, in the skin, is one of the most reliable theories about the link between Th17 homeostatic barrier functions and dysregulation leading to the failure of immunological tolerance, chronic inflammation, and autoimmune disease mediation by Th17 cells [135-139]. Th17 cells have the ability to enhance B-cell responses. This could be further evidence for a role for Th17 cells either directly or through trans-differentiation to Th cells in promoting the production of autoantibodies [140, 141].

Robak et al. [45] found increased mean serum concentrations of IL-17B, IL-17E, and IL-17F in patients with systemic sclerosis and assumed that IL-17 cytokines play a role in its pathogenesis [45]. The literature regarding the role of IL-17A in systemic sclerosis is quite vague. Some studies report an elevated level of IL-17A in SSc, others note no such elevation in the early and late stages of the disease, and no difference was found between dcSSc and lcSSc [33, 62, 143-145]. However, it was shown that measurement of IL-17 is not sensitive enough to give a clear picture of the profile of Th17 lymphocytes in SSc. Chizzolini et al. stated that in patients with SSc, serum levels of IL-17A are generally low [39]. Some studies indicate that IL-17A plays a key role in the early inflammatory stage of the disease, characterized by the predominance of Th1 and Th17 cells. In contrast, in the late stage, Th2 cells are more relevant [33, 62, 142, 143].

The serum concentration of IL-17E was also higher in patients with SSc than in healthy individuals. IL-17E is expressed by a variety of cells, such as CD4+ cells, CD8+ T cells, macrophages, dendritic cells, mast cells, eosinophils, epithelial and endothelial cells [146–153]. IL-17E influences type 2 immunity and inhibits Th17-mediated inflammation [146, 150–154]. Increased numbers of IL-17E+ cells were found in the dermis of both morphea and systemic sclerosis. IL-17E may enhance fibrosis by favoring a Th2-like response, which induces the synthesis of collagen by fibroblasts and induces activated macrophages. [155].

The Crucial Role of the Imbalance of Th17 and Treg Cells in SSc

Pathogenesis of SSc is a complex process that is mediated by multiple cells and their balances, which seem to be more pivotal than structural or molecular deficiencies of single T cell subsets [28]. In addition to the alternation of the canonical Th1/Th2 balance, the imbalance of Th17/Treg has gathered much attention recently.

There are relevancies between the differentiation of Th17 and Treg lineages. TGF-β, a potent regulatory cytokine that maintains tolerance via the regulation of lymphocyte proliferation, differentiation, and survival, has been demonstrated to be required for Foxp3 expression in peripheral naïve T cells [108, 109]. In the presence of TGF-β, antigen-activated naïve T cells express both RORγt, a Th17 lineage-specific transcription factor, and Foxp3, but the function of RORγt is antagonized by Foxp3 [110, 111]. The generation of Th17 cells from such RORγt+Foxp3+ cells requires the presence of IL-6, IL-21, and IL-23, while the differentiation of Treg cells needs IL-2 and retinoic acid [20, 62, 112-115]. IL-6 has various effects and biological activities in immune regulation, hematopoiesis, inflammation, and oncogenesis. As described, at the mutual precursor of Th17 and Treg cells, Foxp3 can inhibit the transcriptional activation of RORγt, leading to the upregulation of Treg cell proliferation. This inhibition can be abolished in the presence of IL- 6, thus promoting the differentiation of Th17 cells [114, 115]. On the other hand, it can be speculated that IL-6 may suppress Treg cell differentiation associated with their alternation [117]. Due to the significant effects of the differentiation of Th17 and Treg cells, IL-6 impacts their balance. In addition, IL-23 has been found to promote the development and expansion of Th17 cells and may be induced by low concentrations of TGF-β, together with IL-6 or IL-21 [115, 118]. Under the influence of those nonnegligible cytokines, Th17 and Treg cells may have a reciprocal relationship through antagonistic competition of Foxp3 and RORγt.

Moreover, some studies suggested that a fraction of Treg cells probably can differentiate into IL-17-producing cells, i.e., Th17 cells due to their cytokine milieu [82, 101, 119–123]. Although these IL-17-producing Treg cells may still maintain the immunosuppressive function, this plasticity of Treg cells results in both pro-inflammation activities and autoimmunity [119, 123]. On the contrary, there seems to be no study that suggested Th17 cell subsets have the same performance differentiating into Treg cells. In addition, Treg cells' plasticity is linked to both gene expression and epigenetic programming [112, 120].

It has been demonstrated that breaking the Th17/Treg balance in peripheral blood may play an important role in the development of autoimmunity-related diseases, including SLE, connective tissue diseases-associated pulmonary arterial hypertension (CTD-aPAH), RA, primary immune thrombocytopenia (ITP), and HIV infections. It has also been associated with the activity and severity of diseases [24, 57, 82, 91, 124-126]. Further, IL-6 could be deduced to mediate the Th17/Treg balance according to its upregulation of Th17 cells, and the suppression of Treg cells since studies about it shows the correlation between SSc activity and disability [127].

There are also studies that have revealed the numerical and functional deficiency of Th17 and Treg cells co-existing in SSc and increased the ratio of Th17/Treg cells, which suggests that the immune response in SSc is skewed towards Th17 cell generation or expansion, leading to the pro-inflammation, fibrosis, and vascular abnormalities [28, 67, 101]. It has also been found that Treg cells with the capacity to secrete IL-17 are involved in SSc [101].

As mentioned above, Th17 cells secrete the IL-17 family, IL-21, IL-22 and other cytokines. They can facilitate the synthesis of collagen and ECM, the migration of dermal vascular smooth muscle cells (DVSMCs), the differentiation of endothelium into myofibroblasts, which might also produce exaggerated amounts of ECM, and they have effects on multiple immunocytes. These activities are closely related to chronic inflammation and fibrosis in the skin, blood vessels, and internal organs in SSc. Normal Treg cells and their products, such as TGF-β, IL-10, and IL-35, maintain immune homeostasis and inhibit the inflammatory process; however, SSc Treg cells, with a numeral or functional abnormalities, could promote the development of adaptive immune responses to autoantigens [128]. Further, Treg cells in SSc turn into Th2-like cells to activate the fibroblasts and upregulate the collagen and ECM deposition [107]. Hence, defective Treg cells in SSc aggravate the inflammatory and fibrotic process that contributes to dermal, vessel, and visceral damage. Therefore, due to the differentiative and functional antagonism of the Th17 and Treg cell lineages, the increased Th17/Treg ratio observed in SSc patients represents the enhancement of Th17 function and the reduction of Treg suppression, which contributes to widespread fibrosis, persistent inflammation, and microangiopathy, and leads to the manifestation of tissue damage in SSc.

There are some studies about the mechanisms of Th17/Treg balance in vivo. Directly regulated by Rbpj protein transcription, Notch signaling in dendritic cells has been identified to participate in the balance of Th17 and iTreg cells [129]. Some researchers found that α-ketoglutaric acid can increase Foxp3 expression and antagonize the function of transcription factor RORγt, in other words, which means it could block the differentiation of Th17 cells and up-regulated Treg cells [130]. It could be speculated that Notch signaling and glutamate-dependent metabolic pathway might participate in Th17/Treg balance, but their roles in SSc pathogenesis needs more experiments to identify.

There is no curative therapy for SSc so far. In consideration of the Th17/Treg imbalance, therapeutic approaches associated with Th17 and Treg cell subsets are in the spotlight, and there is an abundance of hypotheses aimed at Th17 or Treg cells alternation. For instance, since the Th17/Treg balance is skewed towards Th17 cells inhibiting pro-inflammatory cytokines, which drive Th17 differentiation, such as IL-6, IL-1β, and IL-21, they may be more effective in restoring the Th17/Treg balance [131, 132]. As for Th17-associated strategies, treatments that target the key Th17 cytokine production IL-17 pathway are under consideration [133]. In addition, it has been reported that IL-17- and IL-23-specific antibody treatments are effective for some immune-mediated inflammatory diseases, and may also be used for SSc [134].

Th17 and Treg cells are agonistically competitive in their differentiation and function. Antigen-activated naïve T cells express both RORγt and Foxp3 in the presence of TGF-β, and Foxp3 is capable of inhibiting the transcriptional activation of RORγt. Depending upon the local cytokine environment, such as RORγt(+)Foxp3(+) cells differentiate into Th17/Treg cells. In SSc pathogenesis, Th17 cells secrete the IL-17 family, IL-21, IL-22, and other cytokines to promote the synthesis of collagen and ECM, the migration of DVSMCs, the differentiation of endothelium into myofibroblasts, and they have effects on multiple immunocytes. Abnormalities of Treg cells in SSc, such as reduced deficiency, dysfunction, and turning to Th2-like cells, might reduce their immunosuppression of Th17 and other immunocytes and promote the development of autoimmune antibodies. All of the mechanisms above contribute to chronic inflammation and fibrosis in the skin, blood vessels, and internal organs in SSc. Thus, the Th17/Treg cells balance skews towards Th17 cell subsets and causes a series of pathological processes of SSc.

There are an obvious interest and proof about Th17 implication in SSc, but there are still some questions that are not answered. It is not yet clear if Th17 cells have a direct pro-fibrotic action. Also, the fine-tuning between Treg/Th17/Th1/Th2 and maybe other Th subsets is not well described in SSc patients yet. There are promising data that suggest inhibition of Treg and Th1 signals on the one hand and promotion of Th17 and Th2 signals on the other [156]. This fine-tuning could also be a marker for the SSc course, and this interesting aspect needs to be further studied.

CONCLUSION

An aberrant T-cell homeostasis is a crucial event in SSc pathogenesis, and a Th17/Treg imbalance appears to be important. Th17 cells act as effector cells exhibiting their pro-fibrosis and pro-inflammation capabilities, while Treg cells resist the inflammatory and fibrotic process in SSc. Due to their altered immunological behaviors and interaction, an imbalance of Th17 and Treg cells shows a significant impact on SSc pathogenesis.

REFERENCES

[1] Varga J, Maria T, Masataka K. Pathogenesis of systemic sclerosis: recent insights of molecular and cellular mechanisms and therapeutic opportunities, *J. Scleroderma Relat. Disord.* 2017;3-137.

[2] Guiducci S, Distler O, Distler JH, et al. Mechanisms of vascular damage in SSc – implications for vascular treatment strategies. *Rheumatology* (Oxford) 2008;47(Suppl 5):v18–20. doi:10.1093/rheumatology/ken26.

[3] Parel Y, Aurrand-Lions M, Scheja A, et al. Presence of CD4 + CD8+ double-positive T cells with very high interleukin-4 production potential in lesional skin of patients with systemic sclerosis. *Arthritis Rheum.* 2007;56(10):3459–67. doi:10.1002/art.22927.

[4] Barsotti S, Stagnaro C, Della Rossa A. Systemic sclerosis: a critical digest of the recent literature. *Clin Exp Rheumatol* 2015;33:3-14.

[5] Gabrielli A, Avvedimento EV, Krieg T. Scleroderma. *N Engl J Med.* 2009;360:1989–2003. doi:10.1056/NEJMra0806188.

[6] Mo C, Zeng Z, Deng Q, et al. Imbalance between T helper 17 and regulatory T cell subsets plays a significant role in the pathogenesis of systemic sclerosis. *Biomed. Pharmacother.* 2018;108:177-183. https://doi.org/10.1016/j.biopha.2018.09.037

[7] Cabral-Marques O, Riemekasten G. Vascular hypothesis revisited: role of stimulating antibodies against angiotensin and endothelin receptors in the pathogenesis of systemic sclerosis, *Autoimmun. Rev.;* 2016.

[8] Chizzolini C, Brembilla NC, Montanari E, et al. Fibrosis and immune dysregulation in systemic sclerosis. *Autoimmun. Rev.* 2011;10-276.

[9] Lipsky PE. Systemic lupus erythematosus: an autoimmune disease of B cell hyperactivity. *Nat Immunol.* 2001;2(9):764–6.

[10] Lafyatis R, O'Hara C, Feghali-Bostwick CA, et al. B cell infiltration in systemic sclerosis-associated interstitial lung disease. *Arthritis Rheum.* 2007;56(9):3167–8.

[11] Whitfield ML, Finlay DR, Murray JI, et al. Systemic and cell type-specific gene expression patterns in scleroderma skin. *Proc Natl Acad Sci U S A*. 2003;100(21):12319–24.

[12] Sato S, Fujimoto M, Hasegawa M, et al. Altered blood B lymphocyte homeostasis in systemic sclerosis: expanded naive B cells and diminished but activated memory B cells. *Arthritis Rheum*. 2004;50(6):1918–27.

[13] Wang J, Watanabe T. Expression and function of Fas during differentiation and activation of B cells. *Int Rev Immunol*. 1999;18(4):367–79.

[14] Sato S, Hasegawa M, Fujimoto M, et al. Quantitative genetic variation in CD19 expression correlates with autoimmunity. *J Immunol. 1* 2000;65(11):6635–43.

[15] Tsuchiya N, Kuroki K, Fujimoto M, et al. Association of a functional CD19 polymorphism with susceptibility to systemic sclerosis. *Arthritis Rheum*. 2004;50(12):4002–7.

[16] Yoshizaki A, Iwata Y, Komura K, et al. CD19 regulates skin and lung fibrosis via toll-like receptor signaling in a model of bleomycin-induced scleroderma. *Am J Pathol*. 2008;172(6):1650–63.

[17] Matsushita T, Hasegawa M, Yanaba K, et al. Elevated serum BAFF levels in patients with systemic sclerosis: enhanced BAFF signaling in systemic sclerosis B lymphocytes. *Arthritis Rheum*. 2006;54(1):192–201.

[18] Matsushita T, Fujimoto M, Hasegawa M, et al. Elevated serum APRIL levels in patients with systemic sclerosis: distinct profiles of systemic sclerosis categorized by APRIL and BAFF. *J Rheumatol*. 2007;34(10):2056–62.

[19] Bielecki M, Kowal K, Lapinska A, et al. Increased production of a proliferation-inducing ligand (APRIL) by peripheral blood mononuclear cells is associated with antitopoisomerase I antibody and more severe disease in systemic sclerosis. *J Rheumatol*. 2010; 37(11):2286–9.

[20] O'Reilly S, Hugle T, van Laar JM. T cells in systemic sclerosis: a reappraisal, *Rheumatol. Oxf*. (Oxford) 2012;51:1540.

[21] Gizinski AM, Fox DA. T cell subsets and their role in the pathogenesis of rheumatic disease, *Curr. Opin. Rheumatol.* 2014;26:204.

[22] Omoyinmi E, Hamaoui R, Pesenacker A, et al. Th1 and Th17 cell subpopulations are enriched in the peripheral blood of patients with systemic juvenile idiopathic arthritis, *Rheumatol. Oxf.* (Oxford) 2012;51.

[23] Truchetet ME, Brembilla NC, Montanari E, et al. Increased frequency of circulating Th22 in addition to Th17 and Th2 lymphocytes in systemic sclerosis: association with interstitial lung disease, *Arthritis Res. Ther.* 2011;13:R166.

[24] Talaat RM, Mohamed SF, Bassyouni IH, et al. Th1/Th2/Th17/Treg cytokine imbalance in systemic lupus erythematosus (SLE) patients: correlation with disease activity, *Cytokine* 2015;72:146.

[25] Meloni F, Solari N, Cavagna L, et al. Frequency of Th1, Th2 and Th17 producing T lymphocytes in bronchoalveolar lavage of patients with systemic sclerosis, *Clin. Exp. Rheumatol.* 2009;27:765.

[26] Antonelli A, Ferri C, Fallahi P, et al. Th1 and Th2 chemokine serum levels in systemic sclerosis in the presence or absence of autoimmune thyroiditis, *J. Rheumatol.* 2008;35:1809.

[27] Muroi E, Ogawa F, Shimizu K, et al. Elevation of serum lymphotactin levels in patients with systemic sclerosis, *J. Rheumatol.* 2008;35:834.

[28] Fenoglio D, Battaglia F, Parodi A, et al. Alteration of Th17 and Treg cell subpopulations co-exist in patients affected with systemic sclerosis, *Clin. Immunol.* 2011;139:249.

[29] Yoshizaki A, Yanaba K, Iwata Y, et al. Cell adhesion molecules regulate fibrotic process via Th1/Th2/Th17 cell balance in a bleomycin-induced scleroderma model, *J. Immunol.* 2010;185:2502.

[30] Prescott RJ, Freemont AJ, Jones CJ, et al. P. Sequential dermal microvascular and perivascular changes in the development of scleroderma. *J Pathol* 1992;166:255–63. doi:10.1002/path. 1711660307.

[31] Harrison NK, Myers AR, Corrin B, et al. Structural features of interstitial lung disease in systemic sclerosis. *Am Rev Respir Dis* 1991;144:706–13. doi:10.1164/ajrccm/144.3_Pt_1.706.

[32] Singh RP, Hasan S, Sharma S, et al. 17 cells in inflammation and autoimmunity. *Autoimmun Rev* 2014;13:1174–81. doi:10.1016/j. autrev.2014.08.019.

[33] Kurasawa K, Hirose K, Sano H, et al. Increased interleukin-17 production in patients with systemic sclerosis. *Arthritis Rheum* 2000;43:2455–63. doi:10.1002/1529-0131(200011) 43:11-2455:aid-anr12.3.0.co;2-k.

[34] Rodriguez-Reyna TS, Furuzawa-Carballeda J, Cabiedes J, et al. 17 peripheral cells are increased in diffuse cutaneous systemic sclerosis compared with limited illness: a cross-sectional study. *Rheumatol Int* 2012;32:2653–60. doi:10.1007/s00296-011-2056-y.

[35] Fossiez F, Djossou O, Chomarat P, et al. T cell interleukin-17 induces stromal cells to produce proinflammatory and hematopoietic cytokines. *J Exp Med* 1996;183:2593–603. doi:10.1084/jem.183.6. 2593.

[36] Xing X, Yang J, Yang X, et al. IL-17A induces endothelial inflammation in systemic sclerosis via the ERK signaling pathway. *PLoS One* 2013;8:e85032. doi:10.1371/journal.pone.0085032.

[37] Truchetet ME, Brembilla NC, Montanari E, et al. Interleukin-17A+ cell counts are increased in systemic sclerosis skin and their number is inversely correlated with the extent of skin involvement. *Arthritis Rheum* 2013;65:1347–56. doi:10.1002/art.37860.

[38] Lei L, Zhao C, Qin F, et al. 17 cells and IL-17 promote the skin and lung inflammation and fibrosis process in a bleomycin-induced murine model of systemic sclerosis. *Clin Exp Rheumatol* 2016;34(Suppl 100):14–22.

[39] Chizzolini C, Dufour AM, Brembilla NC. Is there a role for IL-17 in the pathogenesis of systemic sclerosis? *Immunol Lett* 2018;195:61–7. doi:10.1016/j. imlet.2017.09.007.

[40] Yang X, Yang J, Xing X, et al. Increased frequency of 17 cells in systemic sclerosis is related to disease activity and collagen overproduction. *Arthritis Res* 2014;16:R4. doi:10.1186/ar4430.

[41] Park M, Moon S, Lee E, et al. IL-1-IL-17 signaling axis contributes to Fibrosis and inflammation inTwo Different Murine Models of systemic sclerosis. *Frontiers in Immunology* 2018;9:1-12 doi: 10.3389/fimmu.2018.01611.

[42] Gourh P, Arnett FC, Assassi S, et al. Plasma cytokine profiles in systemic sclerosis: associations with autoantibody subsets and clinical manifestations. *Arthritis Res* 2009;11:R147.

[43] Olewicz-Gawlik A, Danczak-Pazdrowska A, Kuznar-Kaminska B, et al. Interleukin-17 and interleukin-23: importance in the pathogenesis of lung impairment in patients with systemic sclerosis. *Int J Rheum Dis* 2014;17:664–70.

[44] Kolls JK, Lindén A. Interleukin-17 family members and inflammation. *Immunity 2004*;21:467-76.

[45] Robak E, Gerlicz-Kowalczuk Z, Dziankowska-Bartkowiak B, et al. Serum concentrations of IL-17A, IL-17B, IL-17E and IL-17F in patients with systemic sclerosis. *Arch Med Sci* 2019;15(3):706-712.

[46] Hymowitz SG, Filvaroff EH, YIN JP, et al. IL-17s adopt a cystine knot fold: structure and activity of a novel cytokine, IL-17F, and implications for receptor binding. *EMBO J.* 2001;20:5332–41.

[47] Rodríguez-Reyna TS, Furuzawa-Carballeda J, Cabiedes J, et al. Th17 peripheral cells are increased in diffuse cutaneous systemic sclerosis compared with limited illness: a cross-sectional study. *Rheumatol Int* 2012;32: 2653-60.

[48] Radstake TR, van Bon L, Broen J, et al. The pronounced Th17 profile in systemic sclerosis (SSc) together with intracellular expression of TGFbeta and IFNgamma distinguishes SSc phenotypes. *PLoS One* 2009;4:e5903.

[49] Zhang Z, Xiao C, Gibson AM, et al. EGFR signaling blunts allergen-induced IL-6 production and Th17 responses in the skin and attenuates development and relapse of atopic dermatitis, *J. Immunol.* 2014;192:859.

[50] Camporeale A, Poli V. IL-6, IL-17 and STAT3: a holy trinity in auto-immunity? *Front. Biosci. Landmark Ed* 2012;17:2306.
[51] Singh B, Schwartz JA, Sandrock C, et al. Modulation of autoimmune diseases by interleukin (IL)-17 producing regulatory T helper (Th17) cells, *Indian J. Med. Res.* 2013;138:591.
[52] Kluger MA, Luig M, Wegscheid C, et al. STAT 3 programs Th17-specific regulatory T cells to control GN, *J. Am. Soc. Nephrol.* 2014;25:1291.
[53] Ghoreschi K, Laurence A, Yang XP, et al. T helper 17 cell heterogeneity and pathogenicity in autoimmune disease, *Trends Immunol.* 2011;32:395.
[54] Marwaha AK, Leung NJ, McMurchy AN, et al. TH17 cells in autoimmunity and immunodeficiency: protective or pathogenic? *Front. Immunol.* 2012;3:129.
[55] Chiricozzi A, Zhang S, Dattola A, et al. New insights into the pathogenesis of cutaneous autoimmune disorders, *J. Biol. Regul. Homeost. Agents* 2012;26:165.
[56] Paulissen SM, van Hamburg JP, Dankers W, et al. The role and modulation of CCR6+ Th17 cell populations in rheumatoid arthritis, *Cytokine* 2015;74:43.
[57] Wang W, Shao S, Jiao Z, et al. The Th17/Treg imbalance and cytokine environment in peripheral blood of patients with rheumatoid arthritis, *Rheumatol. Int.* 2012;32:887.
[58] Wilde B, Thewissen M, Damoiseaux J, et al. Th17 expansion in granulomatosis with polyangiitis (Wegener's): the role of disease activity, immune regulation and therapy, *Arthritis Res. Ther.* 2012;14;R227.
[59] Babaloo Z, Aliparasti MR, Babaiea F, et al. The role of Th17 cells in patients with relapsing-remitting multiple sclerosis: interleukin-17A and interleukin-17F serum levels, *Immunol. Lett.* 2015;164;76.
[60] Tuzun E, Huda R, Christadoss P. Complement and cytokine based therapeutic strategies in myasthenia gravis, *J. Autoimmun.* 2011;37:1 36.

[61] Komura K, Fujimoto M, Hasegawa M, et al. Increased serum interleukin 23 in patients with systemic sclerosis, *J. Rheumatol.* 2008;35:120.

[62] Mathian A, Parizot C, Dorgham K, et al. Activated and resting regulatory T cell exhaustion concurs with high levels of interleukin-22 expression in systemic sclerosis lesions, *Ann. Rheum. Dis.* 2012;71:1227.

[63] Zhou Y, Hou W, Xu K, et al. The elevated expression of Th17-related cytokines and receptors is associated with skin lesion severity in early systemic sclerosis, *Hum. Immunol.* 2015;76:22.

[64] Nakashima T, Jinnin M, Yamane K, et al. Impaired IL-17 signaling pathway contributes to the increased collagen expression in scleroderma fibroblasts, *J. Immunol.* 2012;188:3573.

[65] Lonati PA, Brembilla NC, Montanari E, et al. High IL-17E and low IL-17C dermal expression identifies a fibrosis-specific motif common to morphea and systemic sclerosis, *PLoS One* 2014; 9:e105008.

[66] Okamoto Y, Hasegawa M, Matsushita T, et al. Potential roles of interleukin-17A in the development of skin fibrosis in mice, *Arthritis Rheum.* 2012;64:3726.

[67] Papp G, Horvath IF, Barath S, et al. Altered T-cell and regulatory cell repertoire in patients with diffuse cutaneous systemic sclerosis, *Scand. J. Rheumatol.* 2011;40:205.

[68] Lei L, Zhong XN, He ZY, et al. IL-21 induction of CD4+ T cell differentiation into Th17 cells contributes to bleomycin-induced fibrosis in mice, *Cell Biol. Int.* 2015;39:388.

[69] Liu M, Yang J, Xing X, et al. Interleukin-17A promotes functional activation of systemic sclerosis patient-derived dermal vascular smooth muscle cells by extracellular-regulated protein kinases signalling pathway, *Arthritis Res. Ther.* 2014;16:4223.

[70] Brembilla NC, Montanari E, Truchetet ME, et al. Th17 cells favor inflammatory responses while inhibiting type I collagen deposition by dermal fibroblasts: differential effects in healthy and systemic sclerosis fibroblasts, *Arthritis Res. Ther.* 2013;15:R151.

[71] Peng X, Xiao Z, Zhang J, et al. IL-17A produced by both gamma/delta T and Th17 cells promotes renal fibrosis via RANTES-mediated leukocyte infiltration after renal obstruction, *J. Pathol.* 2015;235:79.

[72] Mi S, Li Z, Yang HZ, et al. Blocking IL-17A promotes the resolution of pulmonary inflammation and fibrosis via TGF-beta1-dependent and -independent mechanisms, *J. Immunol.* 2011;187:3003.

[73] Gasse P, Riteau N, Vacher R, et al. IL-1 and IL-23 mediate early IL-17A production in pulmonary inflammation leading to late fibrosis, *PLoS One* 2011;6:e23185.

[74] Li D, Cai W, Gu R, et al. Th17 cell plays a role in the pathogenesis of Hashimoto's thyroiditis in patients, *Clin. Immunol.* 2013;149:411.

[75] Tan Z, Qian X, Jiang R, et al. IL- 17A plays a critical role in the pathogenesis of liver fibrosis through hepatic stellate cell activation, *J. Immunol.* 2013;191:1835.

[76] Zenewicz LA, Flavell RA. Recent advances in IL-22 biology. *Int. Immunol.* 2011;23:159.

[77] Koumakis E, Bouaziz M, Dieude P, et al. A regulatory variant in CCR6 is associated with susceptibility to antitopoisomerase-positive systemic sclerosis, *Arthritis Rheum.* 2013;65:3202.

[78] Park SH, Kim MS, Lim HX, et al. IL-33-matured dendritic cells promote Th17 cell responses via IL-1beta and IL-6. *Cytokine* 2017;99:106.

[79] Ye J, Wang Y, Liu X, et al. TLR7 signaling regulates Th17 cells and autoimmunity: novel potential for autoimmune therapy. *J. Immunol.* 2017;199:941.

[80] He Z, Wang F, Zhang J, et al. Regulation of Th17 differentiation by IKKalpha-dependent and -independent phosphorylation of RORgammat. *J. Immunol.* 2017;199:955.

[81] Wing JB, Sakaguchi S. Foxp3(+) T(reg) cells in humoral immunity, *Int. Immunol.* 2014;26:61.

[82] Abdulahad WH, Boots AM, Kallenberg CG. FoxP3+ CD4+ T cells in systemic autoimmune diseases: the delicate balance between true

regulatory T cells and effector Th-17 cells, *Rheumatol. Oxf.* (Oxford) 2011;50:646.

[83] Miyara M, Gorochov G, Ehrenstein M, et al. Human FoxP3+ regulatory T cells in systemic autoimmune diseases, *Autoimmun. Rev.* 2011;10:744.

[84] Michels-van AJ, Walter GJ, Taams LS. CD4+CD25+ regulatory T cells in systemic sclerosis and other rheumatic diseases, *Expert Rev. Clin. Immunol.* 2011;7:499.

[85] Baraut J, Grigore EI, Jean-Louis F, et al. Peripheral blood regulatory T cells in patients with diffuse systemic sclerosis (SSc) before and after autologous hematopoietic SCT: a pilot study, *Bone Marrow Transplant.* 2014;49:349.

[86] Shevach EM Mechanisms of foxp3+ T regulatory cell-mediated suppression. *Immunity* 2009;30:636.

[87] Alunno A, Bartoloni E, Bistoni O, et al. Balance between regulatory T and Th17 cells in systemic lupus erythematosus: the old and the new. *Clin. Dev. Immunol.* 2012;82:3085.

[88] Alexander T, Sattler A, Templin L, et al. Foxp3+ Helios+ regulatory T cells are expanded in active systemic lupus erythematosus. *Ann. Rheum. Dis.* 2013;72:1549.

[89] Tselios K, Sarantopoulos A, Gkougkourelas I, et al. The influence of therapy on CD4+CD25(high)FOXP3+ regulatory T cells in systemic lupus erythematosus patients: a prospective study. *Scand. J. Rheumatol.* 2015;44:29.

[90] Sollazzo D, Polverelli N, Palandri F, et al. Circulating CD4+CD25-Foxp3+ cells are increased in patients with immune thrombocytepenia. *Immunol. Lett.* 2015;166:63.

[91] Kleczynska W, Jakiela B, Plutecka H, et al. Imbalance between Th17 and regulatory T-cells in systemic lupus erythematosus. *Folia Histochem. Cytobiol.* 2011;49:646.

[92] Cooles FA, Isaacs JD, Anderson AE. Treg cells in rheumatoid arthritis: an update, *Curr. Rheumatol. Rep.*2013;15:352.

54   *Rositsa V. Karalilova*

[93] Shan Y, Qi C, Zhao J, et al. Higher frequency of peripheral blood follicular regulatory T cells in patients with new onset ankylosing spondylitis. *Clin. Exp. Pharmacol. Physiol.* 2015;42:154.

[94] Du W, Shen YW, Lee WH, et al. Foxp3+ Treg expanded from patients with established diabetes reduce Helios expression while retaining normal function compared to healthy individuals. *PLoS One* 2013;8:e56209.

[95] Radstake TR, van Bon L, Broen J, et al. Increased frequency and compromised function of T regulatory cells in systemic sclerosis (SSc) is related to a diminished CD69 and TGFbeta expression. *PLoS One* 2009;4:e5981.

[96] Slobodin G, Ahmad MS, Rosner I, et al. Regulatory T cells (CD4(+)CD25(bright)FoxP3(+)) expansion in systemic sclerosis correlates with disease activity and severity. *Cell. Immunol.* 2010; 261:77.

[97] Kataoka H, Yasuda S, Fukaya S, et al. Decreased expression of Runx1 and lowered proportion of Foxp3(+) CD25(+) CD4(+) regulatory T cells in systemic sclerosis. *Mod. Rheumatol.* 2015; 25:90.

[98] Klein S, Kretz CC, Krammer PH, et al. CD127(low/-) and FoxP3(+) expression levels characterize different regulatory T-cell populations in human peripheral blood. *J. Invest. Dermatol.* 2010;130:492.

[99] Antiga E, Quaglino P, Bellandi S, et al. Regulatory T cells in the skin lesions and blood of patients with systemic sclerosis and morphoea. *Br. J. Dermatol.* 2010;162:1056.

[100] Wang YY, Wang Q, Sun XH, et al. DNA hypermethylation of the forkhead box protein 3 (FOXP3) promoter in CD4+ T cells of patients with systemic sclerosis. *Br. J. Dermatol.* 2014;171:39.

[101] Liu X, Gao N, Li M, et al. Elevated levels of CD4(+) CD25(+)FoxP3(+) T cells in systemic sclerosis patients contribute to the secretion of IL-17 and immunosuppression dysfunction. *PLoS One* 2013;8:e64531.

[102] Ugor E, Simon D, Almanzar G, et al. Increased proportions of functionally impaired regulatory T cell subsets in systemic sclerosis. *Clin. Immunol.* 2017.

[103] Giovannetti A, Rosato E, Renzi C, et al. Analyses of T cell phenotype and function reveal an altered T cell homeostasis in systemic sclerosis. Correlations with disease severity and phenotypes. *Clin. Immunol.* 2010;137:122.

[104] Sather BD, Treuting P, Perdue N, et al. Altering the distribution of Foxp3(+) regulatory T cells results in tissue-specific inflammatory disease. *J. Exp. Med.* 2007;204:1335.

[105] Sanchez RR, Pauli ML, Neuhaus IM, et al. Memory regulatory T cells reside in human skin. *J. Clin. Invest.* 2014;124:1027.

[106] Klein S, Kretz CC, Ruland V, et al. Reduction of regulatory T cells in skin lesions but not in peripheral blood of patients with systemic scleroderma. *Ann. Rheum. Dis.* 2011;70:1475.

[107] MacDonald KG, Dawson NA, Huang Q, et al. Regulatory T cells produce profibrotic cytokines in the skin of patients with systemic sclerosis. *J. Allergy Clin. Immunol.* 2015;135:946.

[108] Chen W, Jin W, Hardegen N, et al. Conversion of peripheral CD4+CD25- naive T cells to CD4+CD25+ regulatory T cells by TGF-beta induction of transcription factor Foxp3. *J. Exp. Med.* 2003;198:1875.

[109] Josefowicz SZ, Lu LF, Rudensky AY. Regulatory T cells: mechanisms of differentiation and function, *Annu. Rev. Immunol.* 2012;30:531.

[110] Zhou L, Lopes JE, Chong MM, et al. TGF-beta-induced Foxp3 inhibits T(H)17 cell differentiation by antagonizing RORgammat function. *Nature* 2008;453:236.

[111] Zhou L, Littman DR. Transcriptional regulatory networks in Th17 cell differentiation. *Curr. Opin. Immunol.* 2009;21:146.

[112] Lee YK, Mukasa R, Hatton RD, et al. Developmental plasticity of Th17 and Treg cells, *Curr. Opin. Immunol.* 2009;21:274.

[113] Capurso NA, Look M, Jeanbart L, et al. Development of a nanoparticulate formulation of retinoic acid that suppresses Th17 cells and upregulates regulatory T cells. *Self* 2010;1:335.

[114] Bettelli E, Carrier Y, Gao W, et al. Reciprocal developmental pathways for the generation of pathogenic effector TH17 and regulatory T cells. *Nature* 2006;441:235.

[115] Zhou L, Ivanov II, Spolski R, et al. IL-6 programs T(H)-17 cell differentiation by promoting sequential engagement of the IL-21 and IL-23 pathways. *Nat. Immunol.* 2007;8:967.

[116] Mangan PR, Harrington LE, O'Quinn DB, et al. Transforming growth factor- beta induces development of the T(H)17 lineage. *Nature* 2006;441:231.

[117] Nish SA, Schenten D, Wunderlich FT, et al. T cell-intrinsic role of IL-6 signaling in primary and memory responses. *Elife* 2014;3: e1949.

[118] Langrish CL, Chen Y, Blumenschein WM, et al. IL-23 drives a pathogenic T cell population that induces autoimmune inflammation. *J. Exp. Med.* 2005;201:233.

[119] Khoury SJ. Th17 and Treg balance in systemic sclerosis. *Clin. Immunol.* 2011;139:231.

[120] Koenen HJ, Smeets RL, Vink PM, et al. Human CD25highFoxp3pos regulatory T cells differentiate into IL-17-producing cells. *Blood* 2008;112:2340.

[121] Du J, Huang C, Zhou B, et al. Isoform-specific inhibition of ROR alpha-mediated transcriptional activation by human FOXP3. *J. Immunol.* 2008;180:4785.

[122] Voo KS, Wang YH, Santori FR, et al. Identification of IL-17-producing FOXP3+ regulatory T cells in humans. *Proc. Natl. Acad. Sci. U. S. A.* 2009;106:4793.

[123] Beriou G, Costantino CM, Ashley CW, et al. IL-17-producing human peripheral regulatory T cells retain suppressive function. *Blood* 2009;113:4240.

[124] Ji L, Zhan Y, Hua F, et al. The ratio of Treg/Th17 cells correlates with the disease activity of primary immune thrombocytopenia. *PLoS One* 2012;7:e50909.

[125] Gaowa S, Zhou W, Yu L, et al. Effect of Th17 and Treg axis disorder on outcomes of pulmonary arterial hypertension in connective tissue diseases, *Med. Inflamm.* 2014;2014:247372.

[126] Chevalier MF, Petitjean G, Dunyach-Remy C, et al. The Th17/Treg ratio, IL-1RA and sCD14 levels in primary HIV infection predict the T-cell activation set point in the absence of systemic microbial translocation. *PLoS Pathog.* 2013;9:e1003453.

[127] Sfrent-Cornateanu R, Mihai C, Balan S, et al. The IL-6 promoter polymorphism is associated with disease activity and disability in systemic sclerosis. *J. Cell. Mol. Med.* 2006;10:955.

[128] Pattanaik D, Brown M, Postlethwaite BC, et al. Pathogenesis of systemic sclerosis, *Front. Immunol.* 2015;6:272.

[129] Zaman TS, Arimochi H, Maruyama S, et al. Notch balances Th17 and induced regulatory t cell functions in dendritic cells by regulating Aldh1a2 expression. *J. Immunol.* 2017.

[130] Xu T, Stewart KM, Wang X, et al. Metabolic control of TH17 and induced Treg cell balance by an epigenetic mechanism. *Nature* 2017;548:228.

[131] Neurath MF, Finotto S. IL-6 signaling in autoimmunity, chronic inflammation and inflammation-associated cancer. *Cytokine Growth Factor Rev. 2011*;22:83.

[132] Tanaka T. Can IL-6 blockade rectify imbalance between Tregs and Th17 cells? *Immunother.* UK 2013;5:695.

[133] van den Berg WB, McInnes IB. Th17 cells and IL-17 a–focus on immunopathogenesis and immunotherapeutics, *Semin. Arthritis Rheum.* 2013;43:158.

[134] Gaffen SL, Jain R, Garg AV, et al. The IL-23-IL-17 immune axis: from mechanisms to therapeutic testing. *Nat. Rev. Immunol.* 2014;14:585.

[135] Bystrom J, Clanchy F, Taher TE, et al. Functional and phenotypic heterogeneity of Th17 cells in health and disease. *Eur J Clin Invest.* 2019;49:e13032. https://doi.org/10.1111/eci.13032.

[136] Wu HJ, Ivanov II, Darce J, et al. Gut-residing segmented filamentous bacteria drive autoimmune arthritis via T helper 17 cells. *Immunity.* 2010;32:815-827.

[137] Lopez P, de Paz B, Rodriguez-Carrio J, et al. Th17 responses and natural IgM antibodies are related to gut microbiota composition in systemic lupus erythematosus patients. *Sci Rep.* 2016;6:24072.

[138] Mueller DL. Mechanisms maintaining peripheral tolerance. *Nat Immunol.* 2010;11:21-27.

[139] Hopp AK, Rupp A, Lukacs-Kornek V. Self-antigen presentation by dendritic cells in autoimmunity. *Front Immunol.* 2014;5:55

[140] Hirota K, Turner JE, Villa M, et al. Plasticity of TH17 cells in Peyer's patches is responsible for the induction of T cell-dependent IgA responses. *Nat Immunol.* 2013;14:372-379.

[141] Pfeifle R, Rothe T, Ipseiz N, et al. Regulation of autoantibody activity by the IL-23-TH17 axis determines the onset of autoimmune disease. *Nat Immunol.* 2017;18:104-113.

[142] Murdaca G, Colombo BM, Puppo F. The role of Th17 lymphocytes in the autoimmune and chronic inflammatory diseases. *Intern Emerg Med* 2011;6:487-95.

[143] Murata M, Fujimoto M, Matsushita T, et al. Clinical association of serum interleukin-17 levels in systemic sclerosis: is systemic sclerosis a Th17 disease? *J Dermatol Sci* 2008;50:240-2.

[144] Dantas AT, Almeida AR, Sampaio MC, et al. Different profile of cytokine production in patients with systemic sclerosis and association with clinical manifestations. *Immunol Lett* 2018;198: 12-6.

[145] Rolla G, Fusaro E, Nicola S, et al. Th-17 cytokines and interstitial lung involvement in systemic sclerosis. *J Breath Res* 2016;10: 046013.

[146] Iwakura Y, Ishigame H, Saijo S, et al. Functional specialization of interleukin-17 family members. *Immunity* 2011;34:149-62.

[147] Yamaguchi Y, Fujio K, Shoda H, et al. IL-17B and IL-17C are associated with TNF-alpha production and contribute to the exacerbation of inflammatory arthritis. *J Immunol* 2007;179:7128-36.

[148] Cai S, Batra S, Langohr I, et al. IFN-gamma induction by neutrophil-derived IL-17A homodimer augments pulmonary antibacterial defense. *Mucosal Immunol* 2016;9:718-29.

[149] Suzukawa M, Morita H, Nambu A, et al. Epithelial cell-derived IL-25, but not Th17 cell-derived IL-17 or IL- 17F, is crucial for murine asthma. *J Immunol* 2012;189:3641-52.

[150] Song X, Qian Y. The activation and regulation of IL-17 receptor mediated signaling. *Cytokine* 2013;62:175-82.

[151] Kang Z, Swaidani S, Yin W, et al. Epithelial cell-specific Act1 adaptor mediates interleukin-25-dependent helminth expulsion through expansion of Lin(−)c-Kit(+) innate cell population. *Immunity* 2012;36:821-33.

[152] Pan G, French D, Mao W, et al. Forced expression of murine IL-17E induces growth retardation, jaundice, a Th2-biased response, and multiorgan inflammation in mice. *J Immunol* 2001;167:6559-67.

[153] Ballantyne SJ, Barlow JL, Jolin HE, et al. Blocking IL-25 prevents airway hyperresponsiveness in allergic asthma. *J Allergy Clin Immunol* 2007;120:1324-31.

[154] Saenz SA, Taylor BC, Artis D. Welcome to the neighborhood: epithelial cell-derived cytokines license innate and adaptive immune responses at mucosal sites. *Immunol Rev* 2008;226:172-90.

[155] Barron L, Wynn TA. Fibrosis is regulated by Th2 and Th17 responses and by dynamic interactions between fibroblasts and macrophages. *Am J Physiol Gastrointest Liver Physiol* 2011; 300:723-8.

[156] Bălănescu P, Bălănescu E, & Bălănescu A. IL-17 and Th17 cells in systemic sclerosis: A comprehensive review. *Romanian Journal of Internal Medicine* 2017;55(4):198-204. doi: https://doi.org/10.1515/rjim-2017-0027.

[157] Krasimirova E, Velikova T, Ivanova-Todorova E, et al. Treg/Th17 cell balance and phytohaemagglutinin activation of T lymphocytes in peripheral blood of systemic sclerosis patients. *World J Exp Med.* 2017;7:84–96. doi: 10.5493/wjem.v7.i3.84.

[158] Krasimirova E, Kyurkchiev D. T helper cells in the immune-pathogenesis of Systemic sclerosis - current trends. *Acta Medical Bulgarica.* 2017;44(1):57-63. https://doi.org/10.1515/amb-2017-0010.

In: Th17 Cells in Health and Disease ISBN: 978-1-53617-152-5
Editor: Tsvetelina Velikova © 2020 Nova Science Publishers, Inc.

Chapter 4

THE ROLE OF TH17 CELLS IN SPONDYLOARTHRITIS

Yuki Nanke[1,], MD, PhD and Shigeru Kotake[2], MD, PhD*

[1]Institute of Rheumatology,
Tokyo Women's Medical University, Tokyo, Japan
[2]Division of Rheumatology,
First Department of Comprehensive Medicine, Saitama, Japan

ABSTRACT

Spondyloarthritis (SpA) is a form of progressive and chronic inflammatory arthritis. SpA has varied clinical features, such as enthesitis, dactylitis, nail dystrophy, uveitis, and osteitis. This leads to physical limitations and reduces the quality of life. The pathophysiology of SpA has not been fully elucidated; however, it has become clear that Th17 cells and the IL17/IL23 pathway play crucial roles. In this chapter, we focus on the pathogenic role of Th17 cells in SpA.

---

[*] Corresponding Author's Email: ynn@twmu.ac.jp.

62   *Yuki Nanke and Shigeru Kotake*

Keywords: IL-17, Th17, spondylitis, sacroiliitis, ankylosing spondylitis, psoriatic arthritis, enthesitis

INTRODUCTION

Spondyloarthritis (SpA) is a form of progressive and chronic inflammatory arthritis [1, 2, 3]. This leads to physical limitations and reduces the quality of life. SpA includes psoriatic arthritis (PsA), axial SpA (ankylosing spondylitis: AS) and nonradiographic axial SpA, enteropathic arthritis, reactive arthritis, and undifferentiated SpA. The clinical features of SpA are spondylitis, sacroiliitis, axial or peripheral arthritis, and enthesitis. Including joint inflammation, the disease affects skin, gut, heart, urological organs, genital organs, and eyes. The etiology of SpA has not been fully elucidated. Based on genetic, experimental and clinical studies, the IL-17 pathway plays a crucial role in the pathogenesis of SpA. The IL-17 family is composed of six members: IL-17A to IL-17F. IL-17A is a proinflammatory cytokine that promotes osteoclastogenesis and angiogenesis. In this chapter, we focus on the pathogenic roles of Th17 cells in enthesitis and joint inflammation of SpA. In addition, we also discuss the pathogenic roles of Th17 cells in AS and PsA.

IL-17 CYTOKINE

The IL-17 family is composed of six members: IL-17A to IL-17F. IL-17A and IL-17F are proinflammatory cytokines that share 50% sequence homology. IL-17A is commonly referred to as IL-17. IL-17A is referred to as cytotoxic lymphocyte antigen 8 (CTLA8). IL-17 is produced by CD4+ and CD8+ T cells, natural killer T (NKT) cells, $\gamma\delta$T cells, mucosal-associated invariant T (MAIT) cells, mast cells, neutrophils, and group 3 innate lymphoid cells (ILC3). IL-17 activates the nuclear factor-(NF-)κB pathway. IL-17 increases the secretion and production of IL-8 and

The Role of Th17 Cells in Spondyloarthritis 63

granulocyte colony-stimulating factor (G-CSF) and activates neutrophils. IL-17 also leads to the secretion of pro-inflammatory cytokines such as IL-6, TNF, and IL-1. IL-17A and IL-17F play important roles in the pathogenesis of SpA.

TH17 CELLS

Th17 cells are a subset of helper T cells that produce IL-17A, IL-17F, IL-21, IL-22, IL-26, and TNFβ. Th17 cells express the transcription factor RAR-related orphan receptor-γδ (RORγδ). IL-23 is necessary for Th17 cell maturation and stabilization.

THE PATHOGENIC ROLES OF TH17 CELLS IN AS

AS is characterized by joint inflammation, leading to the formation of new bone and progressive ankylosis of the spine and sacroiliac joints. AS frequently affects the enthesis, the anatomical zone where tendons and ligaments insert into the bone. HLA-B27 is strongly associated with AS. It has become clear that the IL-23-IL-17 axis plays a crucial role in the pathogenesis in AS based on genomic studies [4, 5], animal models [6, 7], and translational and clinical studies [8-12].

Variants of IL12B are associated with AS and PsA. Based on a genome-wide association study (GWAS), the susceptibility variants in the IL23R locus are associated with altered transcript levels of genes related to the Th17 cell response in AS [13]. Fiorillo M et al. reported that variants in the HLA-B27 region contribute to disease susceptibility [14]. Bowness P et al. demonstrated that HLA-B27 homodimers bind with high affinity to killer cell immunoglobulin-like receptor 3DLS2 (KIR3DL2), which is expressed on IL-17+CD4+ T cells in sera and synovial fluid of AS patients [15]. The misfolding and homodimer formation of HLA-B27 can activate the IL-17-IL-23 axis [16]. The HLA-B27 homodimerization activates the unfolded protein response and increases IL-23 production [17]. HLA-A02 and HLA-B07 are also associated with AS. Variants in the ERAP1/2 loci, and RUNX3 locus are associated with AS and PsA [4, 18]. IL-1R2, ANTXR 2, and signal transducer and activator of transcription 3 (STAT3) have also been reported to be associated with AS [19]. STAT3 is an important regulator of the function and differentiation of IL-17-producing CD4+ T cells.

Sherlock et al. showed that systemic overexpression of IL-23 induced AS-like enthesitis by triggering IL-17 production from noncanonical double-negative T cells residing at the insertion of ligaments to the bone in an animal model [6]. The levels of IL-17 and/ or IL-23 are higher in serum and synovial fluid of AS patients than healthy controls [20, 21]. IL-17+CD4+ T cells are increased in serum and synovial fluid of patients with AS and positively correlated with disease activity [22]. The levels of IL-17+CD8T cells are also elevated in synovial fluid compared with the serum of patients with SpA and also positively correlated with disease activity [23]. Thus, IL-17+CD8T cells may play an important role in inflammation of HLA class I-associated SpA.

Sherlock et al. reported that IL-22 was the dominant effector cytokine in bone remodeling [6]. IL-22 activates STAT 3-dependent osteoblast-mediated bone remodeling [6, 24]. In addition, PGE2 stimulates the differentiation of osteoblasts. Based on a study of IL-17A-deficit mice, Vg6+γδ T cells produce IL-17A and enhance bone regeneration [25]. It has been reported that in active AS patients, there are increased levels of circulating γδT cells that express IL-23R and produce IL-17 [25-27]. In a mouse model, retinoid-related orphan receptor-γ(RORC)+IL-17A-expressing γδT cells accumulated in the enthesis, aortic root, and eye, which are tissue sites commonly affected by SpA [28].

IL-17-producing cells include neutrophils [9], mast cells [10, 29], γδT cells [26], NKT cells [3], MAIT cells [31, 32) and ILCs [33-35], which are increased in AS. IL-17A expressing γδT cells increased in the serum of patients with AS and PsA [26]. Higher frequencies of IL-17+ mucosal-associated invariant T (MAIT) cells are identified in serum and synovial fluid from patients with AS [31, 32]. In AS, the innate immune pathway mediated by mast cells and neutrophils may also be of relevance [9]. By immunostaining, in the synovia of patients with AS, IL-17 not from T cells, but from ILC, it was expressed [10]. ILCs producing IL-17 and IL-22 are expanded in the peripheral blood, synovial fluid, and bone marrow of patients with AS [33]. Increased expression of IL-17 of CD15+ neutrophils was noted in the subchondral bone marrow of the inflamed spine of an AS patient [9]. TNF blocker is effective for reducing inflammation but not structural progression. Secukinumab, anti-IL-17A antibody, shows sustained efficacy and contributes to slow structural progression in AS patients [8]. Taken together, both the innate and adaptive mechanisms and IL-23-IL-17 axis play crucial roles in AS (Figure 1a and b).

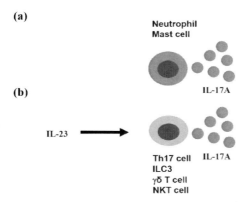

Figure 1. IL-23-independent (a) and dependent (b) production of IL-17A.

BONE METABOLISM OF SpA AND IL-17

One of the characteristic features of SpA is ectopic new bone formation [36]. In SpA, bone formation followed by joint inflammation occurs in the spine (syndesmophytes), at entheses (enthesophytes), and near joints on the periosteal surface (osteophytes). IL-17 enhances the effects of TNF on bone matrix formation by mesenchymal stem cells (MSCs). TNF also induces Dickkopf (Dkk)-1 and sclerostin, both of which block bone formation.

The Wnt/ lipoprotein receptor-related protein (LRP) pathway is critically important for osteoblastic new bone formation. Dkk-1 is an inhibitory molecule involved in regulating the Wnt pathway [37-39]. Daoussis et al. found higher serum DKK-1 levels in AS patients treated with TNF-α blockers than untreated AS patients [40]. TNFα is the main inducer of DKK-1 expression [37]. Dkk-1 blockade leads to complete inhibition of bone erosion and the formation of exuberant osteophytes [37] and elicits axial joint ankylosis [41]. Heiland et al. reported that a high level of functional Dkk-1 predicts protection from syndesmophyte formation in AS [42]. In patients with PsA, Dalbeth et al. reported higher circulating concentrations of Dkk-1 than in healthy controls (HC)[43]. On the other hand, Fassio et al. reported lower levels of Dkk-1 both in new bone formation and bone loss in PsA [41]. There is excessive ectopic ossification in AS; on the other hand, bone destruction and ossification coexist in PsA.

Osteocytes are sensors of bone damage and regulate bone mass. Sclerostin is an osteocyte-specific protein that antagonizes bone morphogenetic protein (BMP) activity and inhibits bone formation. Apple et al. found that serum levels of sclerostin were lower in patients with AS than healthy individuals [44], and low levels of sclerostin were significantly correlated with the formation of new syndesmophytes [44]. Thus, low levels of sclerostin may indicate the onset of new bone formation and be a biomarker for predicting structural progression in AS. Recently, it was reported that serum levels of Dkk-1 and sclerostin increased after treatment with secukinumab, a monoclonal antibody that selectively binds to and neutralizes IL-17A [45].

BMP, a member of the transforming growth factor-β (TGF-β) superfamily, also plays a crucial role in osteoblastogenesis and enthesophyte formation in SpA. BMP 2 and BMP 4 were over-produced in patients with AS [46] and correlated with spinal dysmotility and radiographic scores [46]. SMAD-1 and SMAD-5 were mediated by inflammation and associated with new bone formation for up-regulating the BMP signal. Actually, noggin, an extracellular BMP inhibitor, retards new bone formation [47].

The Role of Th17 Cells in Spondyloarthritis 67

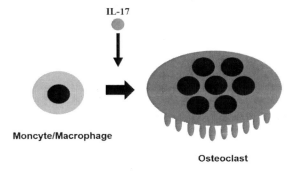

Figure 2. IL-17A potently induces both differentiation and activation of osteoclasts.

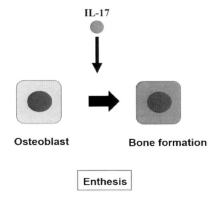

Figure 3. IL-17A induces bone formation of osteoblasts in the enthesis.

IL-17 induces bone destruction by up-regulating the production of matrix metalloproteinase (MMP) and produces receptor activator of nuclear factor kappa-B ligand (RANKL). In RA, IL-17 is associated with bone resorption (Figure 2); on the other hand, in SpA, IL-17 plays a role not only in bone resorption but also in bone formation by enhancing osteoblastogenesis and calcification. IL-17 inhibition reduces both inflammation and new bone formation in experimentally induced SpA [48].

Entheses are key sites of inflammation in SpA; mechanical stress induces bone formation and may also play a pivotal role in the pathogenesis of bone metabolism in SpA patients (Figure 3).

ENTHESITIS AND IL-17

Enthesitis is a hallmark of the clinical features of SpA. Entheses are the insertion sites of ligaments and tendons to bone surfaces and transduce mechanical stress from muscles to bones, and so are essential structures for locomotion. Enthesitis usually occurs outside joints and distant from the synovial joint, and mechanical stress elicits this. Prostaglandin E2 (PGE2) is an important early mediator of enthesitis, and PGE2 induces the production of IL-17 by T cells and activates the IL-23/IL-17 pathway [49].

In studies of animal models, Sherlock et al. showed that IL-23 is essential in the enthesis and acts on an unidentified IL-23 receptor (IL-23R)[+], the RAR-related orphan receptor gt(ROR⁻gt)[+], and stem cell antigen 1 (Sca1)+ entheseal resident T cells [6]. These cells respond to IL-23 and increase the expression of IL-17, IL-6, IL-22, and chemokine (C-X-C motif) ligand 1 (CXCL1) [6, 24]. ILC3 expresses IL-23R and produces IL-17A, which can be seen in human entheses [50].

IL-17 induces neutrophil migration and activation and is associated with IL-23-IL-17 activation, which aggravates enthesitis [6, 51]. IL-23 activating resident T cells in the enthesis promote bone remodeling and inflammation mediated by IL-17 and osteoproliferation mediated by IL-22 [52]. Watad et al. demonstrated the upregulation of IL-17A and evidence for upregulation of IL-17F and IL-22 following the stimulation of human entheseal tissue with IL-23 and IL-1β [53].

The phosphodiesterase 4 inhibitor, apremilast, has been approved for the treatment of PsA. Apremilast inhibits IL-17A, IL-23, and TNF and limits the migration of neutrophils to sites of enthesitis.

THE PATHOGENIC ROLES OF TH17 CELLS IN PSA

Recent studies based on the Classification Criteria for Psoriatic Arthritis (CASPA criteria) indicate that arthritis occurs in up to 30% of patients with psoriasis. It has been reported that in PsA patients, the majority (84%) experience skin symptoms prior to the onset of joint symptoms. Simultaneous onsets of arthritis and psoriatic symptoms occurred in 13% of patients. Only 3% of patients experienced joint involvement preceding skin involvement.

PsA has varied clinical features, such as enthesitis, dactylitis, nail dystrophy, uveitis, and osteitis. TNF-α, IL-17, and IL-23 play crucial roles. TNF-α, transforming growth factor-β, IL-17A and adhesion molecules have been detected in synovia of PsA patients. Immature dendritic cells in PsA show the increased expression of Toll-like receptor2, and this induces a T-helper-1 (Th)-1 cell response with upregulated production of TNF-α, IL-12, and interferon-γ. Activation of the TNF and IL-23-Th17 pathway and pathogenic CD8-positive memory T cells play crucial roles in PsA. Actually, targeting these cells or the pathway has led to successful therapy.

Bone involvement in PsA is heterogeneous. IL-17A induces bone destruction, and IL22 facilitates bone formation. The L-23/IL-17 axis also plays an important role in bone metabolism. It has been reported that in the psoriatic synovium, the receptor activator of NF-κB ligand (RANKL) is upregulated [54]. Moreover, a study showed that osteoclast precursors derived from circulating CD14+ monocytes are markedly elevated in the peripheral blood of patients with PsA [55]. Treatment with anti-TNF agents significantly reduced the level of circulating precursors [55].

IL-17 levels are elevated in PsA skin, synovial tissue, and synovial fluid [56]. Significant enrichment of IL-17+CD4+T cells is present in PsA synovial fluid [57, 58] and synovial tissues [56]. IL-17 induced higher levels of IL-6, IL-8, and MMP-3 production in PsA-fibroblast-like synovial cells (FLS) [56]. IL-17 receptor A (IL-17RA) expression is higher in synoviocytes from patients with PsA than in OA synoviocytes [56]. IL-17+CD8+ T cells are enriched in PsA joints, and numbers are correlated with radiographic erosion [51].

PsA is a highly heritable polygenic disease, and joint involvement occurs in genetically predisposed subjects. HLA alleles and studies of heritability and genome-wide associations have provided evidence that PsA has a genetic component. This is stranger than and distinct from that of psoriasis; it has been reported that HLA-Cw 0602 is associated with psoriasis.

Recent genome-wide association studies of PsA identified certain polymorphisms in the gene encoding IL23R, variants of the TRAF3IP2 gene, encoding Act-1 (nuclear factor κB (NF-κB) activator 1), a key mediator of IL-17 signaling, and, a transcription factor in the RUNX3 gene that promotes CD8+ T cell development. IL-12A, IL-12B, IL-23A, IL-21, and STAT3 are also additional risk alleles.

IL-23 could sustain the differentiation and maintenance of the T helper 17 lineage. IL-23 is composed of two subunits, p19 and p40. IL-12 is composed of p40 and p35. The IL-23 p19 subunit and IL12 p40 subunit are associated with psoriasis and PsA. Ustekinumab, an antibody against the p40 subunit, is more effective for patients with compared with those without HLA-Cw0602. Thus, genetic factors and the IL23/IL-17 pathway play crucial roles in the pathogenesis of psoriasis.

PsA associated with the MHC-1 gene and frequencies of HLA-B08, B27, B38, and B39 have been reported, with specific subtypes including symmetric or asymmetric axial disease, enthesitis, dactylitis, and synovitis. HLA-B27 was reported to be associated with enthesitis, symmetric sacroiliitis, and dactylitis, and HLA-B8 was associated with joint fusion, deformities, asymmetric sacroiliitis, and dactylitis. A large, case-control, genotyping association study identified a PsA-specific variant at the IL23R locus. Single-nucleotide polymorphisms in IL12B, IL23A, IL-23R, and STAT3, whose protein products are involved in the differentiation of Th17 cells, confer susceptibility to PsA. B7-cross-reactive antigen shows cross-reaction with HLA-27. Approximately 25% of patients with PsA are HLA-B27-positive.

IL-17+ CD8+ T cells are enriched in joints of PsA patients and correlated with disease activity and joint damage progression [51]. Mast cells [27], γδ T cells, neutrophils, and MAIT cells [59] have been found in the synovial fluid of PsA patients and produce IL-17. Human mast cells store and release bioactive exogeneous IL-17A [29].

In PsA synovium, marked up-regulation of RANKL and low expression of its antagonist, OPG, have been detected [54]. IL-17-

producing cells accumulate and induce inflammation and upregulate the production of RANKL and then activate osteoclastogenesis.

ILC3s that produce IL-17A and IL-22 have been detected in the peripheral blood [34] and synovial fluid [35] of patients with PsA, they are correlated with disease activity, and show increased expression of CCR6 and potently produce IL-17 [60].

In synovial fluid and synovia of PsA patients, interferon (IFN) γ, IL-2, IL-4, TNF-α, IL-17, and granulocyte-macrophage colony-stimulating factor (G-CSF) are also detected.

The suggestion that Th17 cells play a crucial role in PsA is supported by clinical responses to anti-IL-17A antibodies [11, 61].

IL-22 is a cytokine from the IL-10 family. Activated Th17 and Th22 cell subsets are the major sources of IL-22. Entheseal resident cells such as natural killer (NK) cells and γδ T mast cells [10] produce IL-17 and IL-22 on stimulation by IL-23. IL-22 was elevated in synovial fluid of such patients [62, 63], and anti-TNF therapy reduced elevated IL-22 level in serum and synovial fluid of patients with PsA [63]. In PsA, there were more IL-17+ cells than in psoriasis. On the other hand, IL-22 is more expressed in psoriasis than PsA. In animal models, exogenous IL-23-induced enthesitis [6] and augmented Th17 differentiation lead to psoriasis and synovial-entheseal inflammation [64]. IL-22 has the potential to contribute to pannus formation. IL-22 promotes the osteoblast function by upregulating the expression of pro-osteogenic factors, Wnt and BMP; thus, IL22 is an effector cytokine in bone remodeling of PsA.

THERAPY

TNF inhibitor therapy, etanercept, infliximab, adalimumab, golimumab, and certolizumab pegol are licensed for both AS and PsA. Spontaneous remission of PsA is extremely rare. In an observational trial involving patients treated with TNF agents, the rate of partial remission was 23% [44]. As an anti-IL-17-directed therapy, secukinumab is licensed for AS, with arthritis responses similar to those for TNF inhibitor therapy.

Secukinumab [65] and Ixekizumab [66] have shown efficacy against enthesitis, and both have been approved for PsA patients. Brodalumab, which is directed at IL-17RA and blocks IL-17A signaling, has shown efficacy against PsA. P40 antibody, ustekinumab, directed against the shared subunit of IL-12 and IL-23, is effective for the treatment of psoriasis and PsA [67], although results for the skin are more favorable than those for the joints [33]. Ustekinumab led to marked improvement in enthesitis; this supports an important role of the IL-23/IL-17 axis in enthesitis. The anti-il-23/p19 antibody, guselkumab, now licensed for psoriasis, also showed efficacy in a phase II study of PsA [68, 69].

The sustained efficacy of secukinumab regarding both clinical and radiographic outcomes, which were assessed using the modified stroke ankylosing spondylitis spinal score (mSASSS), was reported [8]. Ustekinumab [70], secukinumab [61, 71], and ixekizumab [72] inhibit radiographic progression in patients with PsA.

CONCLUSION

It is clear that TNF-α plays a crucial role in the pathogenesis of SpA because anti- TNF-α showed significant efficacy for patients with SpA [73]. RA and SpA have different underlying mechanisms. The main feature of RA is synovitis, and TNF-α and IL-17 are involved in the induction of osteoclastogenesis and inflammation and cause the destruction of both articular cartilage and bone. On the other hand, enthesitis and new bone formation are clinical hallmarks of SpA. IL-17 plays roles in enthesitis and ectopic ossification. Non-Th17 cells, including $\gamma\delta$T cells, CD8+T cells, ILC, mast cells, and neutrophils also induce IL-17 by stimulating IL-23. In SpA, all these cells contribute to not only bone resorption but also bone formation by enhancing osteoblastogenesis and calcification. There is excessive ectopic ossification in AS, and bone destruction and ossification coexist in PsA.

In the pathogenesis, the MHC class I gene and ERAP1/2 alter CD8+ T-cell development and differentiation (RUNX3) and/or promote increased IL-23 and /or IL-17 production (IL23, IL23R, and STAT3), which are important; thus, IL-23/IL 17 pathway plays crucial roles.

In SpA, the synovial-entheseal complex is the main lesion, and clinical features are synovitis, osteitis, and enthesitis. It is not fully understood why IL-17 shows different behavior in RA and SpA. Clarifying this will help develop strategies of conventional therapy for SpA.

DISCLOSURE STATEMENT

The authors report no conflict of interest. There was no funding received for this study.

REFERENCES

[1] Nanke Y, Kobashigawa T, Kotake S. Efficacy of methotrexate in the treatment of a HLA-27 positive Japanese patient with reactive arthritis. *Nihon Rinsho Meneki Gakkai Kaishi.* 2010;33(5):283-5.

[2] Kotake S, Nanke Y. Chlamydia-associated arthritis and enteropathic arthritis-two important spondyloarthritides. *Nihon Rinsho Meneki Gakkai Kaishi* 2011;34:121-30.

[3] Nanke Y, Kobashigawa T, Yamanaka H, Kotake S. A case of enteropathic arthritis successfully treated with methotrexate. *Nippon Meneki Gakkai Kaishi* 2016;39(3):219-22.

[4] Evans DM, Spencer CC, Pointon JJ et al. Interaction between ERAP1 and HLA-B27 in ankylosing spondylitis implicates peptide handling in the mechanism for HLA-B27 in disease susceptibility. *Nat Genet.* 2011;43: 761-7.

[5] Cotes A, Hadler J, Pointon JP et al. Identification of multiple risk variants for ankylosing spondylitis through high-density genotyping of immune-related loci. *Nat Genet* 2013;45:730-8.

[6] Sherlock JP et al. IL-23 induces spondyloarthropathy by acting on ROR-γt⁺CD3⁺CD4⁻CD8⁻ entheseal resident T cells. *Nan. Med* 2012; 18:1069-1076.

[7] Romero-Sanchez C et al. Association between Th17 cytokine profile and clinical features in patients with sypondyloarthritis. *Clin Exp Rheumatol* 2011;29:828-834.

[8] Braun J, Baraliakos X, Deodhar A et al. Secukinumab shows sustained efficacy and low structural progression in ankylosing spondylitis: 4-year results from the MEASURE1 study. *Rheumatology* 2019;doi:10.1093.

[9] Apple H, Maier R, Wu P, Scheer R, Hempfing A, Kayser R et al. Analysis of IL-17(+) cells in facet joints of patients with spondyloarthritis suggests that the innate immune pathway might be of greater relevance than the Th17-mediated adaptive immune response *Arthritis Res Ther* 2011;13:R95.

[10] Noordenbos T et al. Interleukin-17 positive mast cells contribute to synovial inflammation n spondyloarthritis. *Arthritis Rheum* 2012; 64:99-109.

[11] Kishimoto M, Taniguchi A, Fujishige A, Kaneko S, Haemmerle S, Porter O et al. Efficacy and safety of secukinumab in Japanese patients with active ankylosing spondylitis: 24-week results from an open-label phase 3 study (MEASURE2-J). *Mod Rheumaol* 2018;3:1-9.

[12] Kampylafka E, d'Oliveira I, Linz C, Lerchen V, Stemmler F, Simon D et al. Resolution of synovitis and arrest of catabolic and anabolic bone changes in patients with psoriatic arthritis by IL-17A blockade with secukinumab: results from the prospective PSARTROS study. *Arthritis Res Ther* 2018;20:153.

[13] Coffre M et al. Combination control of Th17 and Th1 cell functions by genetic variations in genes associated with the interleukin-23

signalling pathway in spondyloarthritis. *Arthritis Rheuma* 2013;65: 1510-1521.

[14] Fiorioll MT, Maragno M, Butler R, Dupuis ML, Sorrentino R. CD8+ T cell autoreactivity to an HLA-B27-restricted self-epitope correlates with ankylosing spondylitis. *J Clin Invest* 2000;106:47-53.

[15] Bowness P et al. Th17 cells expressing KIR3DL2+ and responsive to HLA-B27 homodimers are increased in ankylosing spondylitis. *J Immunol* 2011;186:2672-2680.

[16] Dougados M, Baeten D. Spondyloarthritis. *Lancet* 2011;377 (9783): 2127-2137.

[17] DeLay M et al. HLA-B27 misfoldidng and the undolded protein response augment interleukin-23 production and are associated with Th17 activation in transgenic rats. *Arthritis Rheum* 2009;60:2633-2643.

[18] Apel M et al. Variants in RUNX3 contribute to susceptibility to psoriatic arthritis, exhibiting further common ground with ankylosing spondylitis. *Arthritis Rheum.* 2013;65:1224-1231.

[19] Davidson SI et al. Assocation of STAT3 and TNFRSF1 A with ankylosing spondylitis in Han Chinease. *Ann Rhem Dis* 2011;70:289-292.

[20] Apple H, Maier R, Wu P et al. Analysis of IL-17 (+) cells in facet joints of patients with spondyloarthritis suggests that the innate immune pathway might be of greater releance than the Th17-mediated adaptive immnune response. *Arthritis Res Ther.* 2011; 13:R95.

[21] Romero-Sanchez C et al. Association between Th17 cytokine profile and clinical features in patients with sypondyloarthritis. *CLin Exp Rheumatol* 2011;29:828-834.

[22] Xueyi L et al. Levels of circulating Th17 cells and regulatory T cells in ankylosing spondylitis patients with an inadequated response to anti-TNF-α therapy. *J Clin Immunol* 2013;33:151-161.

[23] Wang C, Liao Q, Hu Y, Zhong D. T lymphocyte subset imbalances in patients contribute to ankylosing spondylitis. *Exp Ther Med* 2015; 9:250-256.

[24] Lories RJ, McInnes IB. Primed for inflammation: enthesis-resident T cells. *Nature Medicine*. 2012. 18;1018-9.

[25] Ono T et al. IL-17-producing gdT cells enhance bone regeneration. *Nature communications*. 2016; 10928.

[26] Kenna TJI, Davidson SI, Duan R et al. Enrichment of circulating interleukin -17-secreting interleukin-23 recptor-positive gd T cells in patients with active ankylosing spondylitis. *Arthritis Rheum*. 2012;64:1420-9.

[27] Noordenbos T, Yeremenko N, Gofita I, van de Sande M, Tak PP, Vamete JD et al. Interleukin-17-positive mast cells contribute to synovial inflammation in spondyloarthritis. *Arthritis Rheum* 2012;64:99-109.

[28] Reinhardt A et al. interleukin-23-dependent gd T cells produce interleukin-17 and accumulate in the enthesis, aortic valve, and ciliary body in mice. *Arthritis Rheum* 2016;68:2476-2486.

[29] Noordenbos T et al. Human mast cells capture, store, and release bioactive exogenous IL-17A. *J Leukoc. Biol* 2016;100:453-462.

[30] Chowdhury A, Chaurasia S, Mishira SK, Aggarwal A, Misra R. IL-17 and IFN-γ producing NK and gd-T cells are preferentially expanded in synovial fluid of patients with reactive arthritis and undifferentiated spondyloarhtirits. *Clin Immunol*. 2017;183:207-212.

[31] Hayashi E et al. Involvement of mucosal-associated invariant T cells in ankylosing spondylitis. *J Rheumatol* 2016;43:1695-1703.

[32] Gracey E et al. IL-17 primes IL-17 in mucosal-associated invariant T (MAIT) cells, which contribute to the Th17-axis in ankylosing spondylitis. *Ann Rheum Dis* 2016;75:2124-2132.

[33] Ciccia F et al. Type 3 innate lymphoid cells producing IL-17 and IL-22 are expanded in the gut, in the peripheral blood, synovial fluid and bone marrow of patients with ankylosing spondylitis. *Ann Rheum Dis*. 2015;74:1739-1747.

[34] Soare A et al. Cutting edge: homeostasis of innate lymphoid cells is imbalance in psoriatic arithritis. *J Immunol* 2018;200:1249-1254.

[35] Leijten E F et al. Brief report:enrichiment of actiater group 3 innate lymphoid cells in psoriatic arthritis synovial fluid. *Arthritis Rhum* 2015;67:2673-2678.

[36] Magrey MN, Khan MA. The paradox of bone formation and bone loss in ankylosing spondylitis:evolving new concepts of bone formation and future trends in management. *Curr Rheumatol Rep* 2017; 19:17.

[37] Diarra D, Stolina M, Polzer K, Zwerina J, Ominsky MS, Dwyer D et al. Dickkopf-1 is a master regulator of joint remodeling. *Nat Med* 2007;13:156-63.

[38] Rossini M, Viapiana O, Idolazzi L et al. High level of Dickkopt-1 is associated with low mineral density and higher prevalence of vertebral fractures in patients with ankylosing spondylitis. *Calcif Tissue Int*. 2015;doi:10.1007?s00223-015-0093-3.

[39] Zou Y-C, Yang X-W, Yuan SG et al. Down regulation of dickkopf-1 enhances proliferation and osteogenic potential of fibroblasts isolated from ankylosing spondylitis patients via the Wnt/β-catenin signaling pathway in vitro. *Connect Tissue Res* 2016;1-12.

[40] Daoussis D, Liossis SNC, Solomou EE, Tsanaktsi A, Bounia K, Karampetsou M et al. Evidence that Dkk-1 is dysfunctional in ankylosing spondylitis. *Arthritis Rheum* 2010;62(1):15-158.

[41] Zhao A, Wang G, Wang Y, Yang J, Wang Y, Zhu J et al. Correlation between magnetic resonance imaging (MRI) findings and the new bone formation factor Dkk-1 in patients with spondyloarthritis. *Clin Rdheumatol* 2019;38:465-475.

[42] Heiland GR, Appel H, Poddubnyy D, Zwerina J, Hueber A, Haibel H et al. High level of functional dickkopf-1 predicts protection from syndesmophyte formation in patients with ankylosing spondylitis. *Ann Rhem Dis* 2012;71:572-574.

[43] Dakbeth N, Pool B, Smith T et al. Circulating mediators of bone remodeling in psoriatic arthritis: implications for disordered osteoclastogenesis and bone erosion. *Artritis Res Ther* 2010;12R164.

[44] Apple H et al. Altered Skeletal Expression of Sclerostin and Its Link to Radiographic Progression in Ankylosing Spondylitis. *Arthritis Rheum* 2009;60:3257-62.

[45] Fassio A, Gatti D, Rossini M, Idolazzi L, Giollo A, Adami P et al. Secukinumab produces a quick increase in WNT signaling antagonistsin patients with psoriatic arthritis. *Clin Exp Rheumatol* 2019;37:127-132.

[46] Chen HA, Chen CH, Lin YJ, Chen PC, Chen WS, Lu CL et al. Association of bone morphogenetic proteins with spinal fusion in ankulosing spondulitis. *J Rheumatol* 2010;37(10):2126-32.

[47] Lories RJ et al. Noggin haploinsufficiency differentially affects tissue responses in destructive and remodeling arthritis. *Arthritis Rheum* 2006;54:1736-1746.

[48] Van Tok MN, van Duivenvoorde LM, Kramer I, Ingold P, Pfister S, Roth L et al. Interleukin -17A inhibit on diminishes inflammation and new bone formation in experimental spondyloarthritis. *Arthritis Rheum* 2019;71(4):612-625.

[49] Paulissen SM et al. Synovial fibroblasts directly induce Th17 pathogenicity via the cyclooxygenase/prostaglandin E2 pathway, independent of IL-23. *J immunol* 2013;191:1364-1372.

[50] Cuthbert R J et al. Froup 3 innate lymphoid cells in human enthesis. *Arthritis Rheumaol* 2017;69:1816-1822.

[51] Menon B, Gullick NF, waler GJ et al. Interleukin-17+CD8+T cells are enriched in the joints of patients with psoriatic arthritis and correlated with disease activity and joint damage progression. *Arthritis Rheum* 2014;66:1272-81.

[52] Kehl AS, Corr M, Weisman MH. Enthesitis:new insights into pathogenesis, diagnostic modalities, and treatment. *Arthritis Rheumatol* (Hoboken, NJ). 2016;68(2):312-232.

[53] Watad A, Cuthbert RJ, Amital H, McGonagle D. Enthesitis: much more han focal insertion point inflammation. *Curr Rheumatol* 2018;20:41.

The Role of Th17 Cells in Spondyloarthritis 79

[54] Ritchlin CT, Haas-Smith SA, Li P, Hicks DG, Schwarz EM. Mechanisms of TNF-alpha- and RANKL-mediated osteoclastogenesis and bone resrption in psoriatic arthritis. *J Clin Invest* 2003;111:821-831.

[55] Anandarajah AP, Schwarz EM, Totterman S et al. The effect of etanercept on osteoclast precursor frequency and enhancing bone marrow oedema in patients with psoriatic arthritis. *Ann Rheum Dis* 2008;67:296-301.

[56] Raychaudhuri S P, Raychaudhuri SK, Genovese MC. IL-17 receptor and its functional significance in psoriatic arthritis. *Mol. Cell Bio Chem.* 2012; 359:419-429.

[57] Leipe J, Gruke M, Dechant C, Reindl C, Kerzendorf U, SchulzeKoops H et al. Role of Th17 cells in human autoimmune arthritis. *Arthritis Rheum* 2010;62:2876-85.

[58] Jandus C, Bioley G, Rivals JP, Dudler J, Speiser D, Romero P. Increased numbers of circulating polyfunctional Th17 memory cells in patients with seronegative spondyloarthritis. *Arthritis Rheum* 2008;58:2307-17.

[59] Teunissen MBM, Yeremenko NG, Beaten DLP et al. The IL-17A-producing CD8+ T cell population in psoriatic lesional skin comprises mucosa-associate invariant T cells and conventional T cells. *J Inves Dermatol* 2014;134:2898-907.

[60] Leijten EF, van Kempen TS, Boes M et al. Enrichment of activated group 3 innate lymphoid cells in psoriatic arthritis synovial fluid. *Arthritis Rheum* 2015;67:2673-78.

[61] Mease P, VD Heijde D, Landewe R et al. Secukinumab improve active psoriatic arthritis symptoms and inhibits radiographic progression:primary results form the randomized, double-blind phase III FUTURE 5 study. *Ann Rheum Dis* 2018;0:1-8.

[62] Fiocco U, Sfriso P, Oliviero F, Roux-Lombard P, Scagliori E, Coxxi L et al. Synovial effucion and synovial fluid biomarkers in psoriatic arthritis to assess intraarticular synovial fluid biomarkers in psoriatic arthritis to assess intraarticular tumor necrosis factor-a blockade in the knee joint. *Arthritis Res Ther* 2010;12:R148.

[63] Mitra A, Raychaudhuri SK, Paychaudhuri SP. Functional role of IL-22 in psoriatic arthritis. *Arthritis Res Ther* 2012;14:R65.

[64] Yang L, Fanok MH, Mediero-Munoz A et al. Augumented Th17 differentiation leads to cutaneous and synovio-entheseal inflammation in a novel model of psoriatic arthritis. *Arthritis Rheumtol* 2018.

[65] McInnes IB, Mease PJ, Ritchlin CT, Rahman P, Gottlieb AB, Kirkham B et al. Secukinumab sustains improvement in signs and symptoms of psoriatic arithritis: 2 year results from the phase 3 FUTURE 2 study. *Rheumatology* (Oxford). 2017;56(11):1993-2003.

[66] Mease PJ, van der Heijde D, Ritchlin CT, Okada M, Cuchacovich RS, Shuler CL, et al. Ixekizumab, an interleukin-17A specific monoclonal antibody, for the treatment of biologic-naïve patients with active psoriatic arthritis: results from the 24-week randomized, double-blind, placebo-controlled and active (adalimumab)-controlled period of the phase III traial SPIRIT-P1. *Ann Rheum Dis.* 2017;76(1);79-87.

[67] Chimenti MS, Ortolan A, lorenzin M, et al. Effectiveness and safety of ustekinumab in naïve or TNF-inhibitors failure psoriatic arthritis patients: a 24-month prospective multicentric study. *Clin Rheumatol* 2018; 37(2):397-405.

[68] Deodhar A, Gottilieb AB, Boehncke WH et al. Efficacy and safety of guselkumab in patients with active psoriatic arthritis: a randomized, double-blind, placebo-controlled, phase 2 study. *Lancet* 2018;391: 2213-24.

[69] Deodhar A et al. *OP218 Efficacy and safety results of guselkumab, an anti-il23 monoclonal antibody, in patients with active psoriatic arthritis over 24 weeks: a phase 2a, randomized, double-blind, placebo-controlled study.* 2017;76:142-143.

[70] Kavanaugh A, Puig L, Gottlieb AB, Ritchlin C, Li S, Wang Y et al. Maintenance of clinical efficacy and radiographic benefit through two years of Ustekinumab therapy in patients with active psoriatic arthritis: results from a randomized, placebo-controlled phase III trail. *Arthriris Care Res* 2015;67(12):1739-1749.

[71] Kamplafka E, d'Oliveira L, Linz C, Lerchen V, Stemmler F, Simon D et al. Resolution of synovitis and arrest of catabolic and anabolic bone changes in patients with psoriatic arthritis by IL-17A blockade with secukinumab: results from the prospective PSARTROS study. *Arthritis Res Ther* 2018;20:153.

[72] Deodhar A, Poddubnyy D, Pacheco-Tena C et al. Efficacy of Ixekizumab in the treatment of radiographic axial spondyloarthritis: 16week of results of a phase 3 randomized, double-blind, placebo controlled trial in patients with prior inadequate response or intolerance to tumor necrosis factor inhibitors. *Arthritis Rheuma* 2018; 71(4):599-611.

[73] Ashany D, Steom EM, Goto R, Goodman SM. The effect of TNF inhibition on bone density and fracture risk and of IL17 inhibition on radiographic progression and bone density in patients with axial spondyloarthritis: a systematic literature review. *Curr Rheumaol* 2019;21:20.

In: Th17 Cells in Health and Disease
Editor: Tsvetelina Velikova

ISBN: 978-1-53617-152-5
© 2020 Nova Science Publishers, Inc.

Chapter 5

ALLERGIC RHINITIS, IL-17 AND THE CONCEPT OF A COMMON RESPIRATORY PATHWAY

Kremena Naydenova[1,], MD, Tsvetelina Velikova[2], MD, PhD and Vasil Dimitrov[1], MD, PhD*

[1]Clinical Center of Allergology, University Hospital Alexandrovska;
Department of internal medicine, Medical University of Sofia,
Sofia, Bulgaria
[2]Clinical Immunology, University Hospital Lozenetz,
Sofia University, Sofia, Bulgaria

ABSTRACT

Inflammation of the upper respiratory tract in patients with allergic rhinitis (AR) may contribute to the inflammation of the lower respiratory airways. Several studies demonstrated the involvement of Th17 cells and IL-17 in the immunological mechanism of AR. It is hypothesized that

---

[*] Corresponding Author's Email: kremenann@gmail.com.

upon Th2 pressure, the inflammatory response in the lungs may lead to a rise in Th17-induced neutrophilic inflammation. Thus, the regulatory role of IL-17A on the Th2 immune response is suggested. However, the findings for IL-17 are bidirectional, and the role of Th17 in AR patients remains unclear. The narrow pathogenetic relationship between the nose and the bronchi and the observed interaction between the two respiratory tracts - upper and lower, suggests that the nose may be considered as an "open window" to the bronchi. Moreover, the confirmed role of Th17 cells and related cytokines in the pathogenesis ensures the niche for developing the new drugs targeting this pathway.

Keywords: allergic rhinitis, allergy, Th17 cells, IL-17, inflammation

INTRODUCTION

In recent years, an increase in the prevalence of allergic diseases was observed. Furthermore, allergic diseases are considered among the most socially important conditions in the world. Changes in the environment - urbanization, increased level of hygiene, severe restriction of infectious and parasitic diseases, industrialization, and air pollution in many countries may explain the growing incidence of allergic respiratory disorders [1]. The basis of the so-called Hygiene hypothesis is linked to the reduced exposure to microorganisms in the early stage of life which may lead to increased allergic sensitization and disease development [2]. It has been estimated that one in five people suffer from an allergic disease - allergic rhinitis, bronchial asthma, atopic dermatitis [3], sometimes affecting every third person.

From an immunological point of view, allergic diseases are caused by impaired immune responses. Studies show that the cause of allergic diseases is the imbalance between two primary T cell clones - type 2 and type 1 that are responsible for the hypersensitivity reactions accomplished by humoral and delayed immune responses. The findings of Mosmann and Coffman for both types of T lymphocytes: CD4 + Th1 and CD4 + Th2 cells assist the understanding of the immunopathogenesis of many immune-mediated diseases by differences in cytokine profile and effector functions of the two subpopulations [4].

T-helper 1 or CD4+ cells produce large amounts of IFN-γ, IL-2, TNF, that are directed to intracellular pathogens, whereas Th2 CD4+ cells produce interleukin 4 (IL-4), IL-5, IL-13 which participate in an immune "allergic" response and protection against parasitic infections. Therefore, the existing concept of balance between Th1/Th2 and its disruption has added to the revealing of the molecular and cellular mechanisms of immune responses involved in several diseases [5].

One of the most common allergic diseases is allergic rhinitis (AR), affecting about 40% of the population [6]. It is a common condition in Bulgaria - around 18.2% of the population [7], with the incidence increasing progressively. The disease is IgE-mediated, a non-infectious, affecting the nasal mucosa after contact with environmental allergens [8]. Although AR is not a life-threatening disease, it significantly impairs patients' quality of life and work capacity [9]. Clinically, the condition is presented with sneezing, watery secretion, itching in the nose, and nose clogging. Conjunctival symptoms are often existing - redness of the eye, burning, itching, and tearing of the eyes due to the existence of the naso-ocular axon reflex, after encountering the same allergens in the presence of atopy. The occurrence of AR requires interaction between environmental factors, the immune system, and genetic predisposition.

The entry of allergens in the airways by the inhalation route leads to hyperreactivity, aggregation of many inflammatory cells - eosinophils, mast cells, and lymphocytes into the upper and lower parts of the respiratory tract. Inflammatory cascade generates gene expression of several mediators leading to local and systemic effects. Uncontrolled inflammation in the upper and lower respiratory tract, as well as in the systemic circulation may lead to poor control of AR with subsequent progression of the disease [10]. In the past, AR was considered as a local inflammatory disease of the nose and paranasal cavities. Continuous ongoing research and current data show that it can be seen as a systemic disease, involving the entire airway [11]. There is a link between allergic inflammation of the upper and lower respiratory tract. Thus, AR may be treated as a first step in the progression of respiratory allergy to asthma [12].

THE CONCEPT OF THE COMMON RESPIRATORY PATHWAY

A number of pieces of evidence support the simultaneous presence of AR and bronchial asthma (BA) and the concept of a common airway. These are their embryological and histological, anatomical and physiological similarities, the existence of naso-bronchial interaction [13], the common inflammation, triggers, and genetic factors, clinical observations, epidemiologic data, and therapeutic management [10, 14]. Evidence from epidemiological studies indicates that nasal symptoms are observed in 78% of asthma patients and 38-40% of AR patients with concomitant BA [15, 16].

There is also a link between allergic inflammation of the lower respiratory airways and their bronchial hyperreactivity. On the one hand, this correlation can be explained by conventional risk factors: common allergens, inflammatory cells, and mediators (cysteinyl leukotrienes, prostaglandins, cytokines), both early and late allergic response, genetic predisposition, etc. There are several possible pathophysiological mechanisms by which AR can lead to inflammation of the lower respiratory tract [11].

There is also a link between the two breathing pathways (the so-called nasobronchial reflex). Exposure to cold air, histamine, or other allergenic extracts on the nasal mucosa may lead to immediate bronchospasm. In patients with AR, the normal protective function of airways is not performed due to nasal obstruction. For this reason, subjects are more prone to the direct "attack" by allergens, viruses, bacteria, pollutants from the air, etc. Inflammation of the upper respiratory tract in patients with AR may contribute to the inflammation of the lower respiratory airways, either directly by the flow of nasopharyngeal secretions (the so-called postnasal drip syndrome) [9] or by the entry of inflammatory mediators into the systemic circulation [14]. Nasal provocation with allergens causes respiratory symptoms and decreased lung function in patients with AR as the number of inflammatory cells and mediators in the systemic circulation increases. This conclusively proves that AR is not an isolated local inflammatory disease of the upper respiratory tract. Many studies indicate the relationship between the two airways. In a cross-sectional survey of Shaaban L. et al. [17], they examined a large group of patients with AR and demonstrated the existence of bronchial hyperresponsiveness of lower airways.

From an immunological point of view, the Th2 immune response is at the root of allergic inflammation. In brief, the inflammatory cascade begins with the following sequence - recognition of the antigen by an antigen-presenting (i.e., dendritic) cell [18, 19]. Dendritic cells present the antigen to the T lymphocytes in regional lymph nodes [20, 15]. Th0 lymphocytes recognize the antigen with their surface receptors and activate [21]. Then, they differentiate into Th1 or Th2 subtype. In healthy subjects, the Th1 cell subtype predominates, whereas, in the nasal mucosa and epithelium of AR patients, Th2 cells prevail. Th1 activation results in the release of IL-2 and 1NFy, whereas the Th2 cytokine profile involves the release of IL-2, IL-3, IL-4, IL-5, IL-9, IL-10 and IL-13, GM-CSF [18, 22]. Th2 cytokines stimulate the synthesis of IgE from plasma cells (via IL-4) [18, 22, 21]. IgE implements mast cell cross-linking and allergen cross-linking, followed by mast cell degranulation and release of inflammatory mediators such as histamine, leukotrienes responsible for vascular dilatation, increased vascular permeability, itching, rhinorrhea, increased contraction of smooth muscles in the airways, mucosal secretion, etc. [6, 9]. IgE e key immunoglobulin involved in the I type of allergic reaction by Coombs and Gell, directed against environmental antigens. This is the well-known mechanism observed in the allergic inflammation when encountering an allergen from the environment.

TH17 CELLS IN THE PATHOGENESIS OF ALLERGIC RHINITIS

In recent years with the discovery of Th17 and regulatory T (Treg) cells, significantly complicated the understanding of the Th1/Th2 paradigm [23] and led to expanding our knowledge on the pathogenesis of AR. Th17-related cytokines can be enlisted as IL-6, TGF-b, IL-23, IL-17A, IL-17F, and IL-22 [24]. The involvement of IL-17 in the tissue damage in several autoimmune diseases has been identified. Th17 are a subtype of T lymphocytes, playing an essential role in inflammatory and autoimmune diseases. RORγt is an crucial nuclear transcription factor discriminating Th17 cells from the other Th subsets. IL-17 was established as a vital effector cytokine secreted by them. This cytokine can also be produced by different types of immune cells, such as macrophages, B-lymphocytes, NK- cells, innate lymphoid cells (ILC) and CD8+ cells [25, 2]. IL-17 has a pro-inflammatory effect, stimulates the production of chemokines such as IL-8 and monocyte chemoattractant protein-1, promotes monocyte and neutrophil migration, encourages IL-6 and IgE formation as a result of local inflammation [27, 28].

Some studies are demonstrating the involvement of Th17 and IL-17 in the immunological mechanism of AR. In a study by Huang et al. [29], Th17/Treg cell-mediated immunity was studied in patients with AR. The results show that the ratio of Th17 cells in the peripheral blood of AR patients is significantly increased, and that of Treg cells is decreased. This suggested that the imbalance between Th17/Treg cells may play an essential role in the pathogenesis and severity of AR. Interestingly, both Th17 and Treg cells are derived from naïve T cells. However, Th17 cells mediate the inflammatory response, whereas Treg cells are related to the immune balance. This antagonism between the two cell subtypes plays a vital role in maintaining the immune homeostasis.

Recent studies have shown that both Th2 and Th17 cells are involved in the pathogenesis of allergic airway inflammation by secreting specific cytokines [30]. The Hoyong Lim study examined the stimulated Th2- and

Th17-immunological response in the lungs after the nasal administration of a fungal protease as an allergen induction. From animal models of allergic airway inflammation, it was found that depletion of antigen-presenting cells in the lungs resulted in a decrease in Th2 and an increase in the Th17 cells. It is hypothesized that upon Th2 pressure, the inflammatory response in the lungs may lead to a rise in Th17-induced neutrophilic inflammation.

In Th2-mediated allergic inflammation, the production of IgE antibodies requires two major signals for switching B cells in producing IgE antibodies. The first is provided by the cytokines IL-4 or IL-13 interacting with B-cell receptors. They convert the signal by activating the Janus family of RAS kinases - JAK1 and JAK3, which lead to phosphorylation of the STAT6 transcriptional regulator. The second signal for IgE switching is the additional stimulation between the CD40 ligand on the T- cell surface with CD40 on the B-cell surface [31]. In the study of Milovanovic, IL-17 is involved in B cell switch, confirming the involvement of Th17 cells in allergic diseases and the phenomenon atopy [32]. Th17 cells produce a large number of other mediators, but IL-17 is involved in the production of IgE.

Another study of Degirmenci et al. 2017 [33] presents the relationship of AR and the interleukins IL-10, IL-17, TGF-β, IFN-γ, IL 22, and IL-35, which can be considered a target for a novel therapeutic approach. Th17 cells as a subpopulation of CD4+ Th cells produce: IL-17A, IL-17F, IL-22, TNF-α, and IL-21 [26]. Th17 cells are related to neutrophil infiltration manifesting in the acute phase of allergic reactions. IL-17 has been considered in some studies as a cytokine contributing to the induction of allergen-specific Th2 cells activation, eosinophil aggregation, and IgE production [34]. Thus, the regulatory role of IL-17A on the Th2 immune response is suggested.

However, the findings for IL-17 are bidirectional, and the role of Th17 in AR patients remains unclear. In this study IL-17 and IL-22 were tested in the role of Th17 cells compared to the neutrophil inflammation. It was shown that both interleukins and TGFb were elevated in patients with AR compared to healthy controls. This result confirmed the increased activity of Th17 cells in symptomatic AR patients with seasonal or persistent disease. The data also demonstrate that Th17 cells and their released cytokines are essential for the immunopathogenesis of AR. In parallel, low levels of IFN-γ were measured, which is seen as an indicator of suppression of the Th1 immune response. The levels of IL-35 (a member of the IL-12 family) whose role is associated with proliferation of Treg cells for inhibition of the immune response and Th17 cells function [34].

Local expression of IL-22 in the nasal mucosa of patients with persistent AR is detected. IL-17A and IL-22 can be used as markers to determine the severity of persistent AR. Expression of IL-22 and IL-17A and their correlation with clinical symptoms in patients with the condition suggest that they are involved in its pathogenesis [35]. In experimental mouse models, the association between IL-17 and eosinophil/neutrophil levels, and their involvement in AR, as well as the therapeutic role of antibodies against IL-17 were observed. Following the administration of anti-IL-17 antibodies, there was demonstrated a marked decrease in the levels of the cells mentioned above, a reduction in Th17 and Th2 immune response, and an increase in Treg response. There was also an improvement in the symptoms of AR. The data obtained suggest that the combination of IL-17/Th17/ Treg plays a vital role in the pathogenesis of AR. These studies can be considered in developing a new therapeutic approach in the treatment of AR [36].

IL-17 A can regulate allergic response at in experimentally induced allergic rhinitis. A study in animal models, including IL-17- deficient mice, showed that IL-17A secreted by Th17 cells definitely plays a role in the pathogenesis of AR. In this study, allergic inflammation was induced by nasal ovalbumin (OVA) administration, resulting in elevated serum IL-17A levels. When stimulated with OVA mice deficient in IL-17 exhibited decreased in two of the symptoms of AR - itching, and sneezing, as compared to the other sensitized with OVA mice group. Mice deficient in IL-17 demonstrated also reduced the accumulation of inflammatory cells such as eosinophils, neutrophils, and mast cells, which indicates that IL-17A takes part in attracting the cells mentioned above in the nasal mucosa. Lowered levels of IL-5 and the specific IgE levels were also observed. This indicates that IL-17A deficiency plays a vital role in the Th2 immune response to AR. IL-17A can be considered and as both positive and negative regulators in the pathogenesis of AR by inhibiting mast cell degranulation and response of Th2 cytokines (IL-4, IL-5, IL-13) and reducing the expression of TNF-α and IL1β [37]. These results further demonstrate that IL-17A can play an essential role in allergic inflammation of the nose by reducing not only Th2-mediated immune response but inhibits the process of inflammation.

Ciprandi et al. [38] examined the correlation between elevated serum levels of IL-17 and the exacerbations of AR during the pollen season. Data showed that the levels of IL-17 in serum were associated with clinical symptoms, use of medication for the AR maintenance, and the number of peripheral blood eosinophils during the pollen season. Therefore, serum IL-17 could be measured as a biomarker for the severity of allergic diseases in patients with AR.

In another study by Ciprandi G. et al. [39] in 2009, the researchers compared cytokine profile and frequency of allergen-specific Th cells, producing IL-17 in patients with AR. The study involved patients who had persistent pollen AR and healthy controls in the pollen season. The secreted cytokines were examined *ex vivo* as peripheral CD4+ T lymphocytes and allergen-specific CD4+ T lymphocytes by flow cytometry. The analysis showed that patients with allergic disease had significantly higher rates of both CD4 + IL17-producing cells, and CD4 + IFNγ + IL17-producing cells compared to healthy controls. This result demonstrates the possible role of Th17 in allergic inflammation during the pollen season in patients with AR. The involvement of Th17 cells in the immune response of the allergic diseases, and specifically in allergic rhinitis, was demonstrated. Furthermore, it was confirmed that Th17 cells contribute to the deterioration of immune homeostasis and disease development [39].

In another study by Tsvetkova-Vicheva et al. [40], a link between Th17 lymphocyte production, IL-17, and bronchial hyperreactivity in patients with AR was investigated. The authors measured high levels of IL-17, IL-4, and IL-13 in patients who are sensitized to several inhalation allergens, suggesting the relationship with allergic rhinitis. The authors did not find a correlation between the bronchial hyperreactivity and IL-17 levels.

The investigated cytology of the nasal mucosa is closely correlated with inflammation of the bronchial mucosa. Due to the close relationship between the upper and lower airways, Sorbello, Ciprandi et al. [41], evaluated Th17 cells and their secreted cytokines - IL-17 A and IL-17 F and the neutrophil count examined in nasal and bronchial biopsy of patients with mild to severe atopic asthma. The results showed predominantly neutrophil phenotype in the severe bronchial asthma and correlation between Th17-related cytokine IL-17F, and to a lesser extent IL-17A in the lamina propria of the nasal and bronchial mucosa. In mild and well-controlled bronchial asthma the increase of IL-17F in bronchial mucosa was less prominent, which suggests a slightly manifested minimal persistent inflammation, dependent on IL-17 levels. Severe BA cases were characterized by more intense IL-17 inflammation in the nasal mucosa than mild BA [41].

Previous studies [42, 43] discussed the similar pathophysiological mechanisms in AR and BA that often occur together. Therefore, the active response of all available therapeutic modalities depends on targeting both diseases simultaneously. The similar pathophysiological mechanism and mucosal inflammation, along with the simultaneous occurrence of AR and BA, suggest the benefit of using the same therapeutic strategy for these patients, including biologic therapy [43].

CONCLUSION

The narrow pathogenetic relationship between the nose and the bronchi and the observed interaction between the two respiratory tracts - upper and lower - suggests that the nose may be considered as an "open window" to the bronchi. Moreover, the confirmed role of Th17 cells and related cytokines in the pathogenesis ensures the niche for developing the new drugs targeting this pathway.

REFERENCES

[1] Kang SY, Song WJ, Cho SH, Chang YS. Time trends of the prevalence of allergic diseases in Korea: A systematic literature review. *Asia Pacific Allergy*. 2018;8(1):e8-e.

[2] Nicolaou N, Siddique N, Custovic A. Allergic disease in urban and rural populations: increasing prevalence with increasing urbanization. *Allergy*. 2005;60(11):1357-60.

[3] Pawankar R, Canonica GW, Holgate ST, Lockey RF, Blaiss MS. *World Allergy Organization (WAO) white book on allergy: update 2013*. Milwaukee (WI): World Allergy Organization; 2013.

[4] Coffman RL. Origins of the TH1-TH2 model: a personal perspective. *Nature Immunology*. 2006;7(6):539-41.

[5] Romagnani S. T-cell subsets (Th1 versus Th2). *Annals of Allergy, Asthma & Immunology*. 2000;85(1):21-18.

[6] Small P, Frenkiel S, Becker A, Boisvert P, Bouchard J, Carr S, et al. Rhinitis: An Executive Summary of a Practical and Comprehensive Approach to Assessment and Therapy. *The Journal of Otolaryngology*. 2007;36(S1):S1.

[7] Mileva F, Popov T, Staneva M, Dimitrov V, et al. Frequency and characteristics of allergic diseases in Bulgaria. *J. Allergy and Asthma*, 2000, Issue 1- Annex, 3-32.

[8] Bousquet J, Khaltaev N, Cruz AA, Denburg J, Fokkens WJ, Togias A, et al. Allergic Rhinitis and its Impact on Asthma (ARIA) 2008 update (in collaboration with the World Health Organization, GA(2)LEN and AllerGen). *Allergy*. 2008;63 Suppl. 86:8-160.

[9] Dykewicz MS, Hamilos DL. Rhinitis and sinusitis. *Journal of Allergy and Clinical Immunology*. 2010;125(2):S103-S15.

[10] Bourdin A, Gras D, Vachier I, Chanez P. Upper airway · 1: Allergic rhinitis and asthma: united disease through epithelial cells. *Thorax*. 2009;64(11):999.

[11] Small P, Keith PK, Kim H. Allergic rhinitis. *Allergy, Asthma & Clinical Immunology*. 2018;14(2):51.

94   *Kremena Naydenova, Tsvetelina Velikova and Vasil Dimitrov*

[12] Kim H, Bouchard J, Renzi PM. The link between allergic rhinitis and asthma: a role for antileukotrienes? *Canadian Respiratory Journal*. 2008;15(2):91-8.

[13] Cingi C, Muluk NB, Cobanoglu B, Çatli T, Dikici O. Nasobronchial interaction. *World Journal of Clinical Cases*. 2015;3(6):499-503.

[14] Caimmi D, Marseglia A, Pieri G, Benzo S, Bosa L, Caimmi S. Nose and lungs: one way, one disease. *Italian Journal of Pediatrics*. 2012;38(1):60.

[15] Simons FER. Allergic rhinobronchitis: The asthma– allergic rhinitis link. *Journal of Allergy and Clinical Immunology*. 1999; 104(3):534-40.

[16] Palma-Carlos AG, Branco-Ferreira M Fau, Palma-Carlos ML, Palma-Carlos ML. Allergic rhinitis and asthma: more similarities than differences. *Allerg. Immunol.* (Paris). 2001 Jun; 33 (6): 237-41.

[17] Shaaban R, Zureik M, Soussan D, Antó JM, Heinrich J, Janson C, et al. Allergic Rhinitis and Onset of Bronchial Hyperresponsiveness. American *Journal of Respiratory and Critical Care Medicine*. 2007;176(7):659-66.

[18] Pawankar R. Inflammatory mechanisms in allergic rhinitis. *Current Opinion in Allergy and Clinical Immunology*. 2007;7 1:1-4.

[19] Roitt I, Brostoff J, Male D. Cell migration and inflammation. *Immunology*. London: Mosby, 1993:13.1-13.8.

[20] Bergeron C, Hamid Q. Relationship between Asthma and Rhinitis: Epidemiologic, Pathophysiologic, and Therapeutic Aspects. *Allergy, Asthma & Clinical Immunology*. 2005;1(2):81.

[21] Male D, Brostoff J, Roth DB, Roitt I. Antigen Presentation. Immunology: Elsevier; 2006. p. 145-62.

[22] Borish L. Allergic rhinitis: Systemic inflammation and implications for management. *Journal of Allergy and Clinical Immunology*. 2003; 112(6):1021-31.

[23] Steinman L. A brief history of TH17, the first major revision in the TH1/TH2 hypothesis of T cell-mediated tissue damage. *Nature Medicine*. 2007;13(2):139-45.

[24] Schmidt-Weber CB, Akdis M, Akdis CA. TH17 cells in the big picture of immunology. *Journal of Allergy and Clinical Immunology*. 2007;120(2):247-54.

[25] Liu Y, Zeng M, Liu Z. Th17 response and its regulation in inflammatory upper airway diseases. *Clinical & Experimental Allergy*. 2015;45(3):602-12.

[26] Miossec P, Korn T, Kuchroo VK. Interleukin-17 and Type 17 Helper T Cells. *New England Journal of Medicine*. 2009;361(9):888-98.

[27] Harrington LE, Hatton RD, Mangan PR, Turner H, Murphy TL, Murphy KM, et al. Interleukin 17-producing CD4+ effector T cells develop via a lineage distinct from the T helper type 1 and 2 lineages. *Nature Immunology*. 2005;6(11):1123-32.

[28] Ivanov II, McKenzie BS, Zhou L, Tadokoro CE, Lepelley A, Lafaille JJ, et al. The Orphan Nuclear Receptor RORgammat directs the differentiation program of proinflammatory IL-17+ T helper cells. *Cell*. 2006;126(6):1121-33.

[29] Huang X, Chen Y, Zhang F, Yang Q, Zhang G. Peripheral Th17/Treg cell-mediated immunity imbalance in allergic rhinitis patients. *Braz. J. Otorhinolaryngol*. 2014;80:152-5.

[30] Lim H, Kim YU, Yun K, Drouin SM, Chung Y. Distinct regulation of Th2 and Th17 responses to allergens by pulmonary antigen presenting cells *in vivo*. *Immunology Letters*. 2013;156(1):140-8.

[31] Janeway CA Jr, Travers P, Walport M, et al. *Immunobiology: The Immune System in Health and Disease*. 5th edition. New York: Garland Science; 2001.

[32] Milovanovic M, Drozdenko G, Weise C, Babina M, Worm M. Interleukin-17A Promotes IgE Production in Human B Cells. *Journal of Investigative Dermatology*. 2010;130(11):2621-8.

[33] Bayrak Degirmenci P, Aksun S, Altin Z, Bilgir F, Arslan IB, Colak H, et al. Allergic Rhinitis and Its Relationship with IL-10, IL-17, TGF-β, IFN-γ, IL 22, and IL-35. *Dis. Markers*. 2018;2018:9131432.

[34] Oboki K, Ohno T, Saito H, Nakae S. Th17 and Allergy. *Allergology International*. 2008;57(2):121-34.

[35] Shahsavan S, Pirayesh A, Samani OZ, Shirzad H, Zamani MA, Amani S, et al. The relationship between IL-17A and IL-22 expression and clinical severity in patients with moderate/severe persistent allergic rhinitis. *American Journal of Otolaryngology.* 2019;40(2):173-8.

[36] Gu ZW, Wang YX, Cao ZW. Neutralization of interleukin-17 suppresses allergic rhinitis symptoms by downregulating Th2 and Th17 responses and upregulating the Treg response. *Oncotarget*; Vol. 8, No 14. 2017.

[37] Quan SH, Zhang YL, Han DH, Iwakura Y, Rhee CS. Contribution of interleukin 17A to the development and regulation of allergic inflammation in a murine allergic rhinitis model. *Annals of Allergy, Asthma & Immunology.* 2012;108(5):342-50.

[38] Ciprandi G, De Amici M, Murdaca G, Fenoglio D, Ricciardolo F, Marseglia G, et al. Serum interleukin-17 levels are related to clinical severity in allergic rhinitis. *Allergy.* 2009;64(9):1375-8.

[39] Ciprandi G, Filaci G, Battaglia F, Fenoglio D. Peripheral Th-17 cells in allergic rhinitis: New evidence. *International Immuno-pharmacology.* 2010;10(2):226-9.

[40] Tsvetkova-Vicheva VM, Gecheva SP, Komsa-Penkova R, Velkova AS, Lukanov TH. IL-17 producing T cells correlate with polysensitization but not with bronchial hyperresponsiveness in patients with allergic rhinitis. *Clinical and Translational Allergy.* 2014;4(1):3.

[41] Sorbello V, Ciprandi G Fau, Di Stefano A, Di Stefano A Fau, Massaglia GM, Massaglia Gm Fau, Favata G, Favata G Fau, Conticello S, Conticello S Fau, Malerba M, et al. Nasal IL-17F is related to bronchial IL-17F/neutrophilia and exacerbations in stable atopic severe asthma. *Allergy* 2015; 70: 236-40.

[42] Velikova Ts, Naydenova K, Dimitrov V. Mucosal Inflammation in Allergic Rhinitis and Bronchial Asthma - Two Sides of a Coin. *Clin. Res. Immunol.* 2018;1(1):1-2.

[43] Naydenova K, Velikova T, Dimitrov V. Interactions of allergic rhinitis and bronchial asthma at mucosal immunology level. *AIMS Allergy and Immunology.* 2019;3(1):1-12.

In: Th17 Cells in Health and Disease
Editor: Tsvetelina Velikova

ISBN: 978-1-53617-152-5
© 2020 Nova Science Publishers, Inc.

Chapter 6

TH17 CELLS IN CHILDHOOD ASTHMA

Snezhina Lazova[1,], MD, PhD, Guergana Petrova[2], MD, PhD and Tsvetelina Velikova[3], MD, PhD*

[1]Pediatric Department,
University Hospital "N. I. Pirogov," Sofia, Bulgaria
[2]Pediatric Clinic, University Hospital Alexandrovska,
Medical University of Sofia, Sofia, Bulgaria
[3]Clinical Immunology, University Hospital Lozenetz,
Sofia University, Sofia, Bulgaria

ABSTRACT

Asthma is a widespread chronic disease characterized by variable and recurrent symptoms, airway obstruction, bronchial hyperreactivity, and underlying inflammation. Airway inflammation in asthma is characterized by the activation of Th2 and Th17 cells, IgE production, and eosinophilia. The involvement of Th17 cells from the early stages of bronchial asthma in children is presented as high percentages of Th17 cells in peripheral blood regardless of disease duration. Although the

---

[*] Corresponding Author's Email: snezhina.lazova@pirogov.bg.

100   *Snezhina Lazova, Guergana Petrova and Tsvetelina Velikova*

mechanism of regulation in cellular and molecular processes that drive the interaction between Th2 and Th17 pathways remains unclear, the data highlight the importance of Th17 immunity in airway inflammation processes. Having in mind the heterogeneity of the disease, targeting Th17/IL-17could help treat patients with the most severe symptoms. However, this should be considered with pronounced caution due to their essential physiological functions in the body.

Keywords: childhood asthma, Th17 cells, IL-17, severe asthma

INTRODUCTION

Asthma is a severe global health problem affecting all age groups, with an incidence of 1-21% in adults and an average of 6-15% in children [1]. According to the World Health Organisation, Global Burden of Disease Study, and the Global Asthma Report, asthma affects nearly 235-334 million people worldwide [2]. In Europe, asthma patients are almost 30 million [3]. Pediatric asthma represents a significant burden for the patient, their family, and the community. It is a leading chronic disease among children in developed countries, affecting five to 20% of school-age children in Europe [51]. The high rate of sleep disturbances due to asthma (up to 34%), school absenteeism (23-51%), and physical activity restriction (47%) have been reported [4]. Asthma is associated with impaired and decreased pulmonary function in childhood. Impairment of lung function at an early age is critical to the future function of the lungs in the adult and significantly increases the risk of chronic obstructive pulmonary disease [5-8]. In most countries, obstructive pulmonary diseases and asthma are the leading cause of visiting emergency centers.

Asthma is a widespread chronic disease characterized by variable and recurrent symptoms, airway obstruction, bronchial hyperreactivity, and underlying inflammation [9-11]. Asthma is a complex syndrome that occurs as a result of exposure to environmental factors such as common allergens, infectious agents, and air pollutants in genetically predisposed individuals and varies in severity, comorbidity, natural history, and therapeutic response [12].

Asthma is also a heterogeneous disease that can be classified into several different phenotypes according to the clinical spectrum of the disease, the inflammatory class, demographic characteristics, and the presence of comorbidity. By definition, the phenotype is a complex of observable features in an organism that results from the interaction of genotype and environmental factors. The asthma-adapted phenotype can be the result of the influence of many factors such as age at onset of asthma symptoms, atopy, inflammatory infiltrate, disease severity, response to standard therapy, etc. [13].

THE ROLE OF TH17 CELLS IN THE PATHOGENESIS OF CHILDHOOD ASTHMA

Bronchial asthma syndrome involves separate subtypes of the disease, which are defined by different pathophysiological mechanisms called endotypes [11]. Among the types of asthma, especially in childhood, allergic asthma is best described and studied. This endotype is characterized by an inflammatory immune response with elevated levels of T helper cell type 2 (Th2) lymphocytes, type 2 lymphoid cells, eosinophils and basophils, together with the activation of tissue-resident cells, in particular epithelial and smooth muscle, leading to hyperproduction of its edema, reversible bronchial obstruction, bronchial hyperreactivity and airway remodeling [13].

The immune response in allergic asthma consists of two main phases - the first phase of sensitization followed by the second effector phase, which can be divided into two sub-phases - 2.1 immediate response and 2.2 late-phase response [14]. Following the discovery of Th1 and Th2 cells in 1986, it has been suggested that the Th2 immune response underlies the development of allergic diseases, whereas the Th1 response predominates in infectious pathology and autoimmunity. CD4+ Th2 cells are established in biopsy material, and lavage fluid (broncho-alveolar lavage, BAL) by patients with allergic asthma and play an essential role in the initiation and development of the disease.

The paradigm for Th2 immune response in asthma explains many of the characteristics of the disease, but there are several observations and features of asthma syndrome that cannot be explained solely by this paradigm. For example, non-Th2 factors such as INFg, neutrophils, and IL-17 are present in the airways of many asthma patients, in particular, those with severe asthma and corticosteroid resistant asthma, confirming that INFg and IL-17 are pro-inflammatory cytokines. There is evidence demonstrating the role of Th1 cells in late-phase exacerbation by inducing apoptosis of the respiratory epithelium of atopic patients [15, 16] and neutralizing IL-17 and IL-17-related effects in experimental asthma models. This leads to a reduction of neutrophils and an increase in eosinophilic infiltration into the lungs [17].

In recent decades, there has been a significant increase in the incidence of both Th1 and Th17 mediated autoimmune conditions (such as DM type 1, IBD, MS) and atopic diseases in Western countries. This, on the one hand, can be explained by an environmentally and lifestyle-influenced change in the function of specific T cell populations with a suppressive capacity called regulatory T cells (Treg), which in turn leads to the development of not only Th2 mediated but also Th1 and Th17 mediated diseases.

The cell subtype secreting large quantities of IL-17A, called Th17 cells, has been identified. Th17 cells play a crucial role in the elimination of extracellular pathogens [18, 19] and are also likely to play a vital role in the development of diseases such as Crohn's disease and rheumatoid arthritis. Several studies with mouse models and humans provide data suggesting the pathogenetic role of Th17 cells in the development of allergic diseases [20, 21]. In humans, Th17 cells play a role in allergic respiratory diseases by inducing smooth muscle cell migration in lower respiratory airways [22].

Due to the variable clinical presentation of childhood asthma, there is a growing scientific and clinical interest in the new asthma phenotypes and endotypes to target individualized therapy [11, 23, 24]. Several childhood pulmonary diseases have immunological mechanisms of development, e.g., pulmonary asthma, allergic rhinitis, cystic fibrosis, etc.

Inhalation of allergens leads to the development of bronchial hyperreactivity as a result of the accumulation of eosinophils, mast cells, and lymphocytes in the wall of the upper and lower respiratory tract and triggering of the inflammatory cascade, generating a local and systemic inflammatory response. Both Th1 and Th2 cells play essential roles in the pathogenesis of allergic rhinitis and bronchial asthma. However, IL-23 dependent Th17 subpopulation that differs from Th1 and Th2 cells and plays a vital role in the inflammation and development of tissue damage in the disease [24, 25].

Although the existence of IL-17 as a product of activated CD4+ T cells has been known for more than ten years, Th17 lymphocytes have been recognized as a distinct subtype of Th cells relatively recently [27, 28]. The IL-17 family is composed of five interleukins, designated as IL-17A to F. IL-17A is homodimeric glycoprotein consisting of 155 amino acids [29], sharing significant homology with IL-17F (55%). IL-17A, as well as IL-17F, may exist as either IL-17A and IL-17F homodimers or IL-17A-IL-17F heterodimers. The primary role of Th17 cells is their ability to recruit and activate neutrophil granulocytes, either directly through the production of IL-8 [30] or indirectly by inducing the production of colony-stimulating factors (CSF) and CXCL8 [31] from tissue cells.

Th17 cells mainly produce IL-17A in distinction from the cytokine profile of CD4+ and CD8+ T cells. Th17 cells are also characterized by activating the nuclear retinoid-coupled orphan receptor (RORγτ). IL-17A overexpression in the lung is observed during acute active neutrophilic inflammation as well as in asthma patients. (4) In some recent studies, the effects of IL-17 and IL-8 on the respiratory epithelium and smooth muscle cells in the bronchial wall have been studied and investigated [27, 28]. Бесидес, effects of IL-17A have been observed, leading to epigenetic alterations, which in turn reduce the ability of corticosteroids to inhibit IL-8 production in human bronchial epithelial cells [29].

104 *Snezhina Lazova, Guergana Petrova and Tsvetelina Velikova*

The balance between Th17 cells and regulatory T cells (Tregs) is critical for maintaining immunological homeostasis. Both the increased number and function of Th17 cells and the decreased number and/or defective function of Tregs can trigger the development and progression of inflammatory diseases, including allergic asthma and allergic rhinitis. Tregs cells express predominantly Forkhead Foxp3 transcription factors that activate many Tregs cell suppressor genes and inhibit many effector T cell genes [26].

Airway inflammation in asthma is characterized by the activation of Th2 cells, IgE production, and eosinophilia. Naïve CD4+ T-helper cells can be induced to differentiate into specific lines of Th1, Th2, Th17, and Treg phenotypes in a mutually exclusive manner. In asthma, an imbalance arises between Th1 and Th2 cells, manifested by an increase in Th2 at the expense of Th1 cells, often due to a decrease in the amount or function of Treg cells [32]. Various pathogens, as well as inflammatory mediators, can impair the suppressive function of T regulatory cells in children with asthma [33]. Moreover, several research teams have described the conversion of Treg cells into a Th17 phenotype by activation of the retinoic acid orphan receptor (RORct) and induction by relevant inflammatory stimuli [34, 35]. IL-17A induces the production of chemokines and antimicrobial peptides from tissue cells, leading to neutrophil accumulation and the development of inflammation [36]. The IL-17 receptor mediates IL-17A activity. IL-17R is expressed by both immune cells and other cells, airway epithelial cells [37]. Considering this, in allergic rhinitis and asthma, IL-17A can cover both innate and adaptive aspects of the immune system, cross-linking the immune system with cells such as airway epithelial cells and fibroblasts [38, 39].

IL-17A is capable of inducing neutrophilic airway inflammation in mice and that this inflammation is insensitive to the action of corticosteroids [40]. Inhaled corticosteroids are the basis of anti-inflammatory treatment for asthma, often used in combination with slow-acting b2-agonists. Managing the treatment of allergic rhinitis and asthma with inhaled corticosteroids is useful in all stages of allergic diseases [41]. Treatment with combination agents is superior to the use of higher doses of inhaled corticosteroids alone [41] and is appropriate to counteract the mechanism of IL-17A mediated inflammation.

In a pharmacogenetic study of Th17 immunity, Albano et al. demonstrated that in children with asthma and allergic rhinitis, Th17 cells more frequently produce IL-17A, confirming their role in systemic and local inflammation and reaffirming the concept of "common airway disease." The results of their study suggest that the potential therapeutic effects of inhaled corticosteroids and slow-acting beta-agonists to control systemic and local inflammation are precisely due to their impact on Th17 immunity in children with allergic respiratory diseases [42].

The results of a study by Cheung et al. indicate that human eosinophils consistently express receptors such as IL-17RA/RC (for IL-17A, F) and IL23R (for IL-23) which stimulate eosinophils to secrete chemokines such as CXCL1, CXCL8, CCL4 and cytokines such as IL-1β, IL-6 and IL-17/IL-23 [43]. IL-17 and IL-23, which are also secreted by dendritic cells and macrophages, affect eosinophilic leukocytes, stimulating the production of cytokines/chemokines, which together with Th17 cells lead to the formation of a vicious circle that indisputably aggravates allergic inflammation [44].

The results of a study by Yamamoto et al. demonstrate the involvement of Th17 cells from the early stages of bronchial asthma in children, evaluating high percentages of Th17 cells in peripheral blood regardless of disease duration [45]. Qing et al. recently conducted a comparative study of Th17 mediated immunological response in children with bronchial asthma. They found that the percentages of circulating Th17 cells and concentrations of Th2- (IL-4, IL-5, and IL-13) and Th17-related cytokines (IL-17A and IL-17E) in plasma are increased in children with allergic diseases compared to non-allergic children or healthy controls [46]. Similar results were reported by Zhao et al., who found that the percentage of Th2 and Th17 cells, as well as the concentration of Th2- and Th17-related cytokines, were higher in asthmatics compared to healthy controls [47].

Studies on the gene expression profile of Th cell genes in the endobronchial tissue of patients with asthma revealed three significant clusters of patients: 1. A group with high Th2 cells; 2. A group with elevated Th17 cells, and 3. A group with low Th2/Th17. When compared with high Th2 cells asthmatics (eosinophil-dominated inflammation), IL-17-related signaling is more demonstrative in the bronchial tissue of the subgroup of patients with moderate to severe asthma [48]. This confirms the assumption that Th17-mediated inflammation may coexist with the Th2 phenotype, enhancing the Th2 response. Patients with an inflammatory model with high IL-5, IL-17A, IL-25 in the respiratory tract often have uncontrolled bronchial asthma [49]. Serum IL-17 levels, on the other hand, are an independent risk factor for the development of severe asthma [50].

Although the mechanism of regulation in cellular and molecular processes that drive the interaction between Th2 and Th17 pathways remains unclear, the data presented above highlight the importance of Th17 immunity in airway inflammation processes. The clinical interpretation of the Th17 inflammatory response and the potential for pharmacological and pharmacogenetic intervention remains to be investigated [51]. On the other hand, understanding the biology of IL-17A can be crucial in developing new therapeutic approaches to overcome the inflammation associated with the cross-link between innate and adaptive immunity during the allergic process in allergic rhinitis and asthma, often insensitive to glucocorticosteroid treatment [42].

Asthma is one of the most common pulmonary diseases in children, but still, the treatment is challenging. The chronic inflammation of the respiratory tract involves T-lymphocytes, IgE-producing plasmocytes, eosinophils, mast cells, macrophages, epithelial cells, fibroblasts and smooth muscle cells of bronchi, and cytotoxic mediators and cytokines (IL-6, IL-8, IL-12, IL-4, IL-10, IL-13, IFN-g, IL-17) [39]. This makes it a complex and heterogeneous disease characterized by intermittent and reversible obstruction and chronic inflammation of the respiratory tract due to bronchial hyperreactivity and infiltration of the respiratory submucosa by immunocompetent cells. The blockage is variable and reversible, spontaneous, or influenced by treatment. There is also an upregulation in the bronchial response to various specific and nonspecific stimuli. About 80% of asthmatics are diagnosed before their 6th year, which proves the early onset of the disease. Furthermore, the natural course is manifested by a progressive decline in respiratory function indicators such as expelled expiratory volume for 1 second, as well as maintaining permanent bronchial hyperreactivity, most likely directly affected by inflammatory and structural changes [25].

Of the T-lymphocytes involved in the pathogenesis of asthma, Th17 lymphocytes are with therapeutic potential. They have shown a critical role in the pathogenesis of nonspecific bronchial reactivity, bronchial asthma, chronic bronchitis, obstructive pulmonary disease, cystic fibrosis, allergic acidosis, allergic acidosis, allergy dermatitis, food allergies, rheumatoid arthritis, systemic lupus, psoriasis, multiple sclerosis, acute respiratory distress syndrome, Crohn's disease, ulcerative colitis, rejection of transplanted kidney, colorectal carcinoma and others [40]. On the other hand, Th17 cells are also involved in the physiological functions of the body, especially the epithelial and mucosal surfaces. In the respiratory tract, they are an intermediate between innate and acquired immunity, playing an essential role in defending the body against extracellular bacteria and fungi by rapidly initiating an acute inflammatory response with a predominant neutrophil involvement. Th17 cells promote effective immune responses and control against bacterial infections, for example P. acnes, C. rodentium, K. pneumoniae, B. pertussis, Bacteroides species, Borrelia species, M. tuberculosis, and some fungi such as C. albicans and others. IL-17 mediated inflammation is characterized by initial irritation by a pathogen or allergen and subsequent differentiation of IL-17 producing cells by naive T lymphocytes. Th17 secreted lymphocyte cytokines (IL-17A, IL-17F, IL-22) induce mucosal and immune cells of innate immunity to secrete a large number of inflammatory cytokines and chemokines that attract locally mast cells, eosinophils and eosinophils enhanced immune responses. The attracted cells, in turn, produce IL-25, which increases Th2 responses and respectively IL-5 and IL-13 secretion. This, in turn, creates the prerequisites for developing asthma or exacerbating the condition. Free oxygen radicals and immune mediators against microbial attacks are involved in tissue damage locally [48].

Not all mechanisms for the involvement of Th17 in the pathogenesis of bronchial asthma have yet been studied, but most literature concludes that in asthma, especially severe, airway inflammation is driven by Th2 along with Th17 lymphocytes. High levels of IL-17 have been found in bronchial-alveolar lavage, serum, and sputum. Irvin et al.'s (2014) study supports the hypothesis that patients with predominantly co-occurrence of Th2 and Th17 lymphocytes are more challenging to treat, have more severe airway obstruction and hyperreactivity [52]. Other researchers have suggested that elevated levels of IL-17 are associated with the severity of hyperreactivity, neutrophil infiltration, exacerbation of asthma, inadequate response to therapy, especially steroids, production of fibrotic mediators, airway remodeling, and pronounced eosinophilia. Increased serum IL-17 marker is an independent risk factor for severe asthma. Thus, without excluding the heterogeneity of the disease, the discovery of new mechanisms in the pathogenesis of the disease could support the treatment of patients with the most severe symptoms [53]. On the other hand, the influence of Th17 cells and their cytokines on childhood asthma should be considered with great care because of their essential physiological functions that they perform in the body.

In chronic obstructive pulmonary disease, some authors have reported increased expression of IL-17 in the bronchial submucosa, while others have not identified one. Our previous studies [54] found that the percentage of Th17 cells is significantly increased in the peripheral blood of children with severe bronchial asthma, especially compared to children with moderate asthma or healthy children. In this way, it was confirmed that particularly in severe asthma, airway inflammation is driven by both Th2 and Th17 cells.

CONCLUSION

Although the mechanism of regulation in cellular and molecular processes that drive the interaction between Th2 and Th17 pathways remains unclear, the data highlight the importance of Th17 immunity in airway inflammation processes. The involvement of Th17 cells from the early stages of bronchial asthma in children is presented as high percentages of Th17 cells in peripheral blood regardless of disease duration.

Having in mind the heterogeneity of the disease, targeting Th17/IL-17 could help treat patients with the most severe symptoms. However, this should be considered with pronounced caution due to their essential physiological functions in the body.

REFERENCES

[1] Lai CK, Beasley R, Crane J, et al. Global variation in the prevalence and severity of asthma symptoms: Phase Three of the International Study of Asthma and Allergies in Childhood (ISAAC) *Thorax* 2009;64(6):476-83.

[2] Innes A. *The Global Asthma Report 2014*. Auckland, New Zealand: Global Asthma Network, 2014 Auckland, New Zealand.

[3] *The European Severe Asthma Servey*, 2005 (Internet).

[4] Fuhlbrigge AL, Guilbert T, Spahn J, et al. The influence of variation in type and pattern of symptoms on assessment in pediatric asthma. *Pediatrics* 2006;118(2):619-25.

[5] Galobardes B, Granell R, Sterne J, et al. Childhood wheezing, asthma, allergy, atopy, and lung function: different socioeconomic patterns for different phenotypes. *Am J Epidemiol.* 2015;182(9):763-74.

[6] Sears MR, Greene JM, Willan AR, et al. A longitudinal, population-based, cohort study of childhood asthma followed to adulthood. *N Engl J Med.* 2003(349):1414-22.

[7] Stern DA, Morgan WJ, Wright AL, et al. Poor airway function in early infancy and lung function by age 22 years: a non-selective longitudinal cohort study. *Lancet.* 2007(370):758-64.

[8] Svanes C, Sunyer J, Plana E, et al. Early life origins of chronic obstructive pulmonary disease. *Thorax.* 2010;65(1):14-20.

[9] Custovic A, Johnston SL, Pavord I, et al. EAACI position statement on asthma exacerbations and severe asthma. *Allergy.* 2013;68(12): 1520-31.

[10] Apter AJ Advances in adult asthma diagnosis and treatment in 2012: potential therapeutics and gene-environment interactions. *J Allergy Clin Immunol.* 2013;131:47-54.

[11] Lotvall J, Akdis CA, Bacharier LB, et al. Asthma endotypes: a new approach to classification of disease entities within the asthma syndrome. *J Allergy Clin Immunol.* 2011;127(2):355-60.

[12] Holt PG, Macaubas C, Stumbles PA, et al. The role of allergy in the development of asthma. *Nature.* 1999;402(6760 Suppl):B12-7.

[13] Oscar Palomares, Cezmi A. Akdis. Chapter 28 Immunology Of the Asthmatic Response, in *Pediatric Allergy Principles and Practice Thir Edition*, Elsevier, 2016, Section F, 250 p,

[14] Larche M, Akdis CA, Valenta R Immunological mechanisms of allergen-specific immunotherapy. *Nat Rev Immunol.* 2006;6(10):761-71.

[15] Trautmann A, Akdis M, Kleemann D, et al. T cell-mediated Fas-induced keratinocyte apoptosis plays a key pathogenetic role in eczematous dermatitis. *J Clin Invest.* 2000;106(1):25-35.

[16] Basinski TM, Holzmann D, Eiwegger T, et al. Dual nature of T cell-epithelium interaction in chronic rhinosinusitis. *J Allergy Clin Immunol.* 2009;124(1):74-80.e1-8.

[17] Hellings PW, Kasran A, Liu Z, et al. mInterleukin-17 orchestrates the granulocyte influx into airways after allergen inhalation in a mouse model of allergic asthma. *Am J Respir Cell Mol Biol.* 2003;28(1):42-50.

[18] Conti HR, Shen F, Nayyar N, et al. Th17 cells and IL-17 receptor signaling are essential for mucosal host defense against oral candidiasis. *J Exp Med.* 2009;206(2):299-311.

[19] Dunne A, Ross PJ, Pospisilova E, et al. Inflammasome activation by adenylate cyclase toxin directs Th17 responses and protection against Bordetella pertussis. *J Immunol.* 2010;185(3):1711-9.

[20] Palomares O, Yaman G, Azkur AK, et al. Role of TREGin immune regulation of allergic diseases. *Eur J Immunol*. 2010; 40(5):1232-40.

[21] Schmidt-Weber CB, Akdis M, Akdis CA TH17 cells in the big picture of immunology. *J Allergy Clin Immunol*. 2007;120(2):247-54.

[22] Chang Y, Al-Alwan L, Risse PA, et al. TH17 cytokines induce human airway smooth muscle cell migration. *J Allergy Clin Immunol*. 2011;127(4):1046-53.e1-2.

[23] Bousquet J AJ, Auffray C, et al. MeDALL (Mechanisms of the Development of ALLergy): an integrated approach from phenotypes to systems medicine. *Allergy*. 2011(66):596-604.

[24] Spycher BD SM, Kuehni CE. Phenotypes of childhood asthma: are they real? *Clin Exp Allergy*. 2010;40:1130–41.

[25] Lazova S. Clinical value of the lung function tests and the atopic status determination in asthmatic children, *2017, MU Sofia, Dissertation*.

[26] L. Cosmi, F. Liotta, E. Maggi, et al. Th17 cells: new players in asthma pathogenesis. *Allergy*. 2011;66(8):989-98.

[27] Oppmann B, Lesley R, Blom B, et al. Novel p19 protein engages IL-12p40 to form a cytokine, IL-23, with biological activities similar as well as distinct from IL-12. *Immunity*. 2000;13(5):715-25.

[28] Cua DJ, Sherlock J, Chen Y, et al. Interleukin-23 rather than interleukin-12 is the critical cytokine for autoimmune inflammation of the brain. *Nature*. 2003;421(6924):744-8.

[29] Yao Z, Fanslow WC, Seldin MF, et al. Herpesvirus Saimiri encodes a new cytokine, IL-17, which binds to a novel cytokine receptor. *Immunity*. 1995;3(6):811-21.

[30] Kullberg MC, Jankovic D, Feng CG, et al. IL-23 plays a key role in Helicobacter hepaticusinduced T cell-dependent colitis. *J Exp Med*. 2006;203(11):2485-94.

[31] Doodes PD, Cao Y, Hamel KM, et al. Development of proteoglycan-induced arthritis is independent of IL-17. *J Immunol*. 2008;181 (1):329-37.

[32] Ghoreschi K, Laurence A, Yang XP, et al. Generation of pathogenic T(H)17 cells in the absence of TGF-b signaling *Nature*. 2010;467 (7318):967-71.

[33] Oukka M. Th17 cells in immunity and autoimmunity. *Ann Rheum Dis* 2008; 67(Suppl 3):26–29.

[34] Kleinschek MA, Boniface K, Sadekova S, et al. Circulating and gut-resident human Th17 cells express CD161 and promote intestinal inflammation. *J Exp Med*. 2009;206(3):525-34.

[35] Santarlasci V, Maggi L, Capone M, et al. TGF-beta indirectly favors the development of human Th17 cells by inhibiting Th1 cells. *Eur J Immunol*. 2009;39(1):207-15.

[36] Gately MK, Renzetti LM, Magram J, et al. The interleukin-12/interleukin-12-receptor system: role in normal and pathologic immune responses. *Annu Rev Immunol*. 1998;16:495-521.

[37] McGeachy MJ, Chen Y, Tato CM, et al. The interleukin 23 receptor is essential for the terminal differentiation of interleukin 17-producing effector T helper cells in vivo. *Nat Immunol*. 2009; 10(3): 314-24.

[38] Fouser LA, Wright JF, Dunussi-Joannopoulos K, et al. Th17 cytokines and their emerging roles in inflammation and autoimmunity. *Immunol Rev*. 2008;226:87-102.

[39] van Beelen AJ, Teunissen MB, Kapsenberg ML, et al. Interleukin-17 in inflammatory skin disorders. *Curr Opin Allergy Clin Immunol*. 2007;7(5):374-81.

[40] Chen Z, O'Shea JJ. Th17 cells: a new fate for differentiating helper T cells. *Immunol Res*. 2008;41(2):87-102.

[41] Kullberg MC, Jankovic D, Feng CG, et al. IL-23 plays a key role in Helicobacter hepaticusinduced T cell-dependent colitis. *J Exp Med*. 2006;203(11):2485-94.

[42] Albano GD, Di Sano C, Bonanno A, et al. Th17 immunity in children with allergic asthma and rhinitis: a pharmacological approach. *PLoS One*. 2013;8(4):e58892.

[43] Cheung, PF, Wong, CK, Lam, CW. Molecular mechanisms of cytokine and chemokine release from eosinophils activated by IL-

17A, IL-17F, and IL-23: implication for Th17 lymphocytes-mediated allergic inflammation. *J Immunol.* 2008;180(8):5625-35.

[44] Koga, C., Kobashima, K., Shiraishi, et al. Possible pathogenic roles of Th17 cells for atopic dermatitis. *J Invest Dermatol.* 2008;128(11): 2625-30.

[45] Yamamoto Y, Negoro T, Wakagi A, et al. Participation of Th17 and Treg Cells in Pediatric Bronchial Asthma. *Journal of Health Science.* 2010;56(5):589–97.

[46] Qing M, Yongge L, Wei X, et al. Comparison of Th17 cells mediated immunological response among asthmatic children with or without allergic rhinitis. *Asian Pac J Allergy Immunol.* 2019;37(2):65-72.

[47] Zhao Y, Yang J, Gao YD, et al. Th17 immunity in patients with allergic asthma. *Int Arch Allergy Immunol.* 2010;151(4):297-307.

[48] Choy DF, Hart KM, Borthwick LA, et al. TH2 and TH17 inflammatory pathways are reciprocally regulated in asthma. *Sci Transl Med.* 2015;7(301):301ra129.

[49] Seys SF, Grabowski M, Adriaensen W, et al. Sputum cytokine mapping reveals an 'IL-5, IL-17A, IL-25-high' pattern associated with poorly controlled asthma. *Clin Exp Allergy.* 2013;43(9):1009-17.

[50] Agache I, Ciobanu C, Agache C, et al. Increased serum IL-17 is an independent risk factor for severe asthma. *Respir Med.* 2010;104(8): 1131-7.

[51] Dimitrova D, Youroukova V. Severe asthma: definition, Immuno-logical characterization And molecular-targeted therapy. *Thoracic Medicine.* 2015;7 (2) :9-25.

[52] Irvin C, Zafar I, Good J, et al. Increased frequency of dual-positive TH2/TH17 cells in bronchoalveolar lavage fluid characterizes a population of patients with severe asthma. *J Allergy Clin Immunol.* 2014;134(5):1175-1186.e7.

[53] Lynch JP, Ferreira MA, Phipps S Th2/Th17 reciprocal regulation: twists and turns in the complexity of asthma phenotypes. *Ann Transl Med*. 2016; 4(Suppl 1): S59.

[54] Velikova T, Lazova S, Perenovska P, et al. Th17 cells in Bulgarian children with chronic obstructive lung diseases. *Allergol Immunopathol* (Madr). 2019;47(3):227-233.

In: Th17 Cells in Health and Disease
Editor: Tsvetelina Velikova

ISBN: 978-1-53617-152-5
© 2020 Nova Science Publishers, Inc.

Chapter 7

TH17 CELLS AND CYSTIC FIBROSIS

Guergana Petrova[1,], Snezhina Lazova[2] and Tsvetelina Velikova[3]*

[1]Pediatric Clinic, University Hospital Alexandrovska,
Medical University of Sofia, Sofia, Bulgaria
[2]Pediatric department, University Hospital "N. I. Pirogov",
Sofia, Bulgaria
[3]Clinical Immunology, University Hospital Lozenetz,
Sofia University, Sofia, Bulgaria

ABSTRACT

Cystic fibrosis (CF) is the most common autosomal recessive life-limiting condition in the Caucasian population. Although the disease is due to established mutations in the CFTR gene, it was shown that Th7 cells and 17 cell–associated cytokines are presented and involved in the lymphocyte-predominant inflammation in the CF lung. Moreover, in the CF airway submucosa, chronic pulmonary inflammation is associated with the stimulation by pathogens such as P. aeruginosa. The excessive attraction of neutrophils in the airways, along with Th17 cells and

---

[*] Corresponding Author's Email: gal_ps@yahoo.co.uk.

cytokines such as IL-17A and IL17F, were shown to be involved in the induction of mucin production, the hyper-contractibility of the airway smooth muscle cells and the corticosteroid resistant airway inflammation in experimental models. We also reviewed the data on macrolides' effect on immunity and especially on Th17 cells and related cytokines production in CF patients.

A more profound understanding of the IL-17-related pathways in the context of CF lung disease is critical to assess the potential implications of anti-IL-17 therapy or interventions targeting its cellular source.

Keywords: Th cells, Th17 cytokines, IL-17, cystic fibrosis, mucoviscidosis

INTRODUCTION

Cystic fibrosis (CF) is the most common life-limiting autosomal recessive condition in the Caucasian population. It is well recognized but less common in other ethnic groups [1]. Average life expectancy has increased from a few years to the mid-30s, with a projected life expectancy for current newborns into the 40s, and if the same trend is preserved, it is expected to reach 70s in the near future [2]. The disease is resulted by malfunctioning protein caused by mutations in the gene encoding the CFTR (cystic fibrosis transmembrane conductance regulator) protein. The protein is an anion channel expressed on the epithelial surface [3]. CFTR dysfunction leads to epithelial cell vulnerability and dysregulation of the local inflammatory responses, which causes excessive airway neutrophilic inflammation and pathogen growth [4]. Thus, CF is typified by the presence of chronic upper and lower respiratory tract infections leading to bronchiectasis and end-stage lung disease. In CF, morbidity and mortality are due primarily to the progressive structural injury and functional decline of the respiratory system [5]. Respiratory symptoms are the leading cause of death in CF. Besides the lung involvement, prominent manifestations also occur in the pancreas, gastrointestinal tract, skin, and male reproductive tract.

Even in cases with absent respiratory symptoms at an early age, airway neutrophilic inflammation has been widely documented, and in many CF patients, it is associated with bacterial colonization. Elevated concentrations of pro-inflammatory cytokines and free neutrophil elastase, peroxidases and oxidants have been consistently found in bronchoalveolar lavage [6]. Initially the bacterial colonization is predominantly *Haemophilus influenzae* and *Staphylococcus aureus*, but with the disease progression and persistent infection, the germs destructing the lung are most notably *Pseudomonas aeruginosa*, and to a lesser extent *Burkholderia cepacia complex*, *Achrombacter xylosoxidans*, *Stenotrophomonas maltophilia* and *Nontuberculous mycobacteria (NTM)* [7-11].

EXCESSIVE INFLAMMATORY RESPONSE AND BACTERIAL INFECTION IN CYSTIC FIBROSIS AIRWAYS

In the CF airways due to CFTR malfunction, there is a reduced chloride secretion and an increase in sodium absorption, which leads to a reduction of the thickness of the periciliary layer, increased mucus volume, and viscosity. This pathogenic cascade is in the foundation of the impairment in the efficacy of the mucus ciliary escalator - a primary airway defense mechanism. Thus it sets up a vicious self enhanced cycle from abundant bacterial growth and powerful inflammatory reaction [12, 13]. Recruitment and activation of inflammatory cells occur with a disproportionate neutrophils influx, that releases proteolytic enzymes, and reactive oxygen species, overwhelm protective mechanisms and cause airway injury and remodeling [4]. Additionally, the increased mucus viscosity impairs neutrophil motility and favors the chronicity of bacterial infection [14, 15]. A simplified overview of the airway inflammatory processes triggered by a microbial infection in CF patients is shown in Figure 1.

Colonization with *P. aeruginosa* results in antibody response, and this normal immune reaction was widely used as a diagnostic tool [16, 17].

However, this response, even very potent is not protective [18]. In contrast, as it was published in 1988, very important for the host defense in CF is the cell-mediated immunity to this pathogen [19].

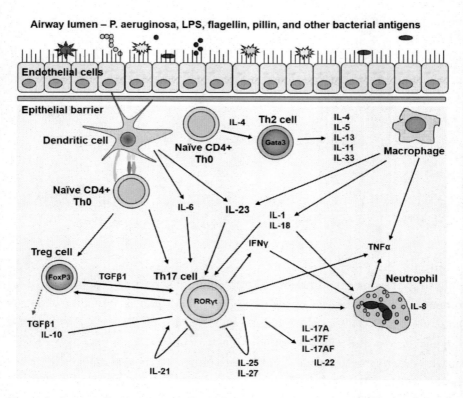

Figure 1. A streamlined summary of the airway inflammatory processes triggered by microbial infections and the central role of Th17 cells in cystic fibrosis patients. Not all mediators and cell types implicated in CF are shown.

Once *P. aeruginosa* is established within the airway, it is almost impossible to be eradicated, as it was shown by genetic studies [20]. Higher antibody titer against *P. aeruginosa* indicates chronic infection and involvement of the immune system. The bacteria produce cilia-toxins, which further impairs ciliary clearance [21]. It also produces proteases that cause tissue damage and cleave immunoglobulins, which further impairs the humoral host response to the organism [22, 23]. These proteases also inhibit the function of phagocytic cells, natural killer cells, and T-lymphocytes by affecting the CD4 molecule on T-helper cells and inhibiting interleukin 1 and interleukin 2 activity [4]. Numerous researches had focussed on CF immunity mainly to T-cells. Recently, attention has been paid on the relatively novel T helper 17 (Th17) subset of Th cells [24].

T-CELL IMMUNITY IN CYSTIC FIBROSIS

CFTR is found not only in epithelial cells. It has been reported to be expressed on lymphocytes [25]; therefore, Mulchay et al. have hypothesized that impaired ion transport resulting from defective CFTR alters T cell responses to antigen stimulation. This alteration may manifest as peripheral changes in the relative proportions of different CD4+ T cell subsets [26]. The authors suggest this idea due to the required ion influx for differentiation, activation, and maturation of the effector T cells after encountering the antigen [26].

T cell-mediated immune responses in people with CF have been reported to be biased towards either T helper (Th)2- or Th17-dominated responses [27]. Notable entity for CF is allergic bronchopulmonary aspergillosis, where a high prevalence of Th2-mediated inflammation was confirmed [28, 29]. Another growing problem in CF is the increasing global incidence and prevalence of NTM infection. CF patients with active M. abscessus complex infection or a history of such showed a distinctive T cell phenotype and a significant deficiency in TNFα production during mitogen stimulation. So far, initial data suggest an association between T cell signatures and individuals at risk of M. abscessus complex infection [30].

Additionally, the finding of the abundancy of Th17 cells and their respective cytokines in airways or lung-draining lymph nodes from people with CF supports the concept for CF as Th17 disease [31].

Th17 Cells and Cystic Fibrosis

In CF, the neutrophilic inflammation prevails in the airway lumen, in the contrast of the lymphocytes predominance in the airway wall. On the genetic level, it was reported that T cells and macrophages have low levels of CTER expression. Thus it was hypothesized that adaptive immunity plays an essential role in the chronic inflammatory process in CF [27].

It was reported that there are varying alterations in the proportions of FOXP3+ Treg, Th17, mucosal-associated invariant T (MAIT) cells, and changes in the relative production of many cytokines in peripheral blood of people with CF [32-34]. Earlier studies have demonstrated the presence of T17 cells - related cytokines such as IL-17 and IL-23, and lymphocyte-predominant inflammation in the CF airway submucosa and lungs of CF patients [35]. Additionally, Tan et al. have confirmed the presence of submucosal Th17 (CD4+IL-17+) lymphocytes in children with CF [36].

Subsequently, Chan and colleagues postulated the need to monitor closely Th17 levels in CF patients on a lung transplant list and follow-up the transplantation, as Th17 has been implicated in transplant rejection [31].

One of the proposed models for the involvement of Th17 cells in pulmonary inflammation is associated with the stimulation by pathogens. *P. aeruginosa* induces the synthesis of IL-6 and IL-23. Together with TGFβ1, the cytokine milieu pushes the differentiation of naive T cells to Th17.

When it was found that Th17% is strongly inversely correlated with lung function (FEV1% predicted) in people with CF one of the hypothesis was that this correlation could be related to the decreasing lung function in CF patients with increasing age, but such significant association was not confirmed, although more changes were noted in adult population compared to the pediatric one [26].

So far, there is no available information about the relative homing to lung and periphery of Th17 cells, but more data had been found that high levels of Th17 cells in the peripheral blood reflect very high levels of Th17 cells locally in the lung [36] and thus, peripheral Th17%, as well as Th17 cells from bronchoalveolar lavage, could be used as a marker of the lung damage.

Another possible explanation for FEV1%pred correlation to Th17% lines in the reported finding for CF high systemic Th17% predisposes to the acquisition of chronic *P. aeruginosa* infection [37]. Such chronic infection is connected with rapid FEV1%pred decline [38], as it was confirmed that patients with chronic *P. aeruginosa* have 2-3 times higher risk for a death in the next eight years compared to the non-chronically infected ones [39]. There are some publications regarding the inability of CF patients to clear *P. aeruginosa* due to abnormalities in the airway surface mucus and ciliary function (as described above), which lead to persisting activation of inflammatory pathways that promote the development of Th17 phenotype and continuous IL-17 production [40]. The excessive attraction of neutrophils in the airways, along with Th17 cells and cytokines such as IL-17A and IL17F, were shown to be involved in the induction of mucin production, the hyper-contractibility of the airway smooth muscle cells and the corticosteroid resistant airway inflammation in mouse models [41].

High percentages of peripheral Th17 cells may be related to an individual's inherent predisposition towards Th17-dominated responses, similar to the susceptibility to Th2 allergic reactions formed very early in life [42-44]. If this is the case, then peripheral blood Th17% was suggested to be beneficial as a prognostic marker of the likelihood of *P. aeruginosa* infection and rapid lung function decline in CF. Velikova et al. have found that pediatric CF patients with isolated *P. aeruginosa* showed higher percentages of Th17 cells than those with no infection [45]. This finding is under the discovery of Tiringer and colleagues for IL-17A as a favorable prognostic marker for infection with *P. aeruginosa* as the levels of IL-17A were higher in CF bronchoalveolar lavage fluid compared with nonCF control subjects [37]. A well-known fact is that Th17 cells are the primary source of IL-17. The same research group has found that IL-17A levels increase even further in CF lung during a pulmonary exacerbation. This elevation was also mirrored by increases in IL-1b and IL-6. These changes correlated with severe decline of FEV1 and additional changes in imaging studies in patients with *P. aerugionasa* infection.

Another research group had proven that CF-knock out mice (without functional CFTR) had defective clearance of the Aspergillus fumigatus, despite a more intense and persistent inflammatory response in the lungs [46]. One week after the infection with the pathogen, the Th17 cytokines (IL-23, IL-17A, and IL-17F) started to increase and were associated with reduced Treg production. The Th17/Treg imbalance was attributed to decreased indoleamine 2,3-dioxygenase levels, the rate-limiting enzyme in tryptophan metabolism. The study demonstrated that the therapies designed to increase tryptophan metabolism (i.e., IFN-g, cyclosporine A, or kynurenines) restored the Th17/Treg imbalance. Therefore, the idea for a possible therapeutic option in these patients by modulating T cell phenotypes and increasing Treg activity was suggested. However, it has to be noted that modulating Th17 responses could lead to higher susceptibility to infections with *Staphylococcus aureus* and *P. aeruginosa* [47]. Therefore so far the most accepted therapeutic approach fighting the chronic inflammation in CF lung is still an aggressive antimicrobial therapy and, to a lesser extent use of anti-inflammatory drugs.

MACROLIDES USE AND IMMUNITY

The macrolides are antibiotics used to treat infections caused by intracellular bacteria, a wide range of gram-positive ones, and limited for gram-negative ones. Thus their utility in CF patients as antibiotics is limited. In addition to their antibiotic activity soon after their introduction in the 1950s, their immunomodulatory properties were also noted [48]. A decade later, a new concept of using macrolides primarily for their immunomodulatory activities was introduced [49]. The immunomodulatory effects were used initially in ophthalmology, urology and general surgery [50]. A crucial for their use in pulmonology was the report of Kudoh and colleagues that erythromycin in adults with diffuse panbronchiolitis leads to dramatically improved survival independent of bacterial colonization [51]. These results encouraged researchers to focus on the use of macrolides for the treatment of other chronic lung diseases as asthma, CF and non-Cf bronchiectasis [52-54]. Clinically the beneficial effects of macrolides as improved symptom scores, stabilizing the lung function, and decreased frequency of exacerbations in COPD and CF have been confirmed with meta-analyses of randomized controlled trials [55, 56].

The immunomodulatory effects have been described using the recommended dose for antimicrobial treatment. Macrolides have excellent tissue penetration with concentrations in macrophages that are 400- to 800-fold higher compared to serum for clarithromycin and azithromycin and 5- to 100-fold higher in tissue compared to serum for erythromycin, clarithromycin, and azithromycin [57-59]. The drug accumulation in immune cells over time may result in immunomodulatory effects occurring even at lower doses and for an extended period compared to the classical antimicrobial effects, which could be tested with future studies. Immunomodulatory effects of macrolides depend on the presence and phase of inflammation. The reported data show that macrolides promote host defenses when administered early during bacterial infection, whereas they inhibit inflammation and promotes its resolution— with potentially adverse effects on defenses—when administered after inflammation has been present for a long time [60].

Aside from ribosomal-mediated inhibition of pathogen (antimicrobial effect), the not related to antimicrobial actions of macrolides range from alterations in cell counts and function, up- and downregulation of cytokine production and expression of adhesion molecules [61]. There is substantial evidence that the immunomodulatory effects macrolides are exerted through inhibition of neutrophilic inflammation and macrophage activation. One of the reported immunomodulatory effects of macrolides is reduced neutrophilic inflammation. This one is based on the usage in neutrophilic asthma, CF, non-CF bronchiectasis, and COPD. The reduced numbers of neutrophils and inhibition of their function (macrolides inhibit the neutrophil release of IL-1β, IL-6, IL-10, TNF-α, CCL1, CCL3, CCL5, CCL20, and CCL22) lead to decreased concentrations of neutrophil elastase and IL-8, and respectively less damage for the lung tissue. Besides neutrophilic inflammation, macrolides also diminish monocytes and macrophages (by increasing phagocytosis and attenuating the secretion of IL-12 by macrophages) triggered inflammation response by decreasing the IL-1beta concentrations. These effects are proven to be due to macrolides' ability to alter intracellular signaling mainly through the inhibition of NF-kappaB activation and expression of activator protein-1 [62-64].

Some studies have reported the macrolides'effect on eosinophilic inflammation as decreased eosinophil counts, and concentration of ECP [65]. Macrolides have a stronger impact on Th2 response (by reducing more frequently Th2 cytokines like IL-4 and IL-5) than on Th1 cytokines (IL-2 and INF-gamma) [66-70].

Immunomodulatory effects likely vary between different macrolides with clarithromycin to have the weakest potency, but so far, none of the human studies directly compared different macrolides. *In vitro* studies have demonstrated that roxithromycin inhibits the chemokine-induced chemotaxis of Th1 and Th2 cells, but not to Treg ones. This effect was not confirmed with clarithromycin and erythromycin [71]. Azithromycin only from this group inhibits IL-1alpha and IL-1beta production [72]. Erythromycin has more potent effect than clarithromycin on reducing IL-6 production by human macrophages [73].

The most studied macrolide for its immunomodulatory effects is azithromycin. Wuyts and colleagues in their *in vitro* study with mice confirmed that azithromycin reduces pulmonary fibrosis. The authors found preservation in pulmonary function tests and decreased fibrosis on histology (reducing the spindle cell proliferation in 60% and 45% decrease in collagen I deposition) in azithromycin-treated mice. As previously noted, the azithromycin effect was observed with the reduction of the neutrophils and lymphocytes when adding azithromycin. Another finding from the study showed that the increase in TH2 and TH17 and decrease of iTreg-related cytokines in bleomycin-treated mice was blocked by the addition of azithromycin [74]. The excessive activation of the TH17 cells plays a role in many diseases characterized by immune dysregulation (inflammatory bowel disease, rheumatoid arthritis, psoriasis, multiple sclerosis, transplantation rejection) [75, 76]. The modulation of the adaptive immune system by azithromycin seems to be by targeting TH1/TH2 fate as well as TH17/iTreg lineage [74].

Besides the effect on immunological cells, azithromycin has shown to reduce inflammation and to modulate host defenses by interacting with structural cells such as epithelial cells, smooth muscle cells, and fibroblasts [77]. The drug reduces mucin secretion and assures the integrity and transepithelial resistance against the permeability induced by *P. aeruginosa* virulence factors in epithelial cells [78, 79]. For the airway smooth muscle cells azithromycin relaxes pre-contracted cells and inhibits IL-17-induced IL-8 [76, 80]. The drug also attenuates fibroblast growth factors induced vascular endothelial growth factor via p38(MAPK) signaling [81]. Additionally, it was confirmed that azithromycin could affect cell autophagy and apoptosis and regulate the expression of several genes involved in mucin production and lipid metabolism [77].

MACROLIDES USE AND CYSTIC FIBROSIS

Knowing that bacteria maintain the chronic inflammatory response, therapies directed towards the chronic infection in CF should reduce inflammation. As mentioned above, azithromycin is the macrolide antibiotic believed to have the most potent anti-inflammatory effects. Besides the potentially positive impact of sub-inhibitory concentrations on *P. aeruginosa*, the drug may benefit CF patients by favorably alter the immune system response against infections and, above all, by alleviating the inflammatory response [56].

Saiman and colleagues confirmed that long term thrice-weekly use of azithromycin in CF patients, who were infected with *P. aeruginosa*, is associated with better lung (improved lung function, decreased exacerbation rates and stabilization of sputum neutrophil elastase) and nutritional (better weight gain) health as well as and quality of life [82]. Similar effects besides the lung function were also found in patients without *P. aeruginosa* infection [83]. In the last two decades, numerous studies and randomized clinical trials have supported the beneficial effect of the long term (over six months) use of azithromycin for CF patients [84]. In the Cochrane review, azithromycin significantly: improved FEV1 over six months compared with placebo (4 studies, n = 549; mean difference 3.97% of predicted, 95% confidence interval [CI] 1.74 to 6.19); improved the rate of being free from exacerbations over 6 months (4 studies, n = 609; odds ratio [OR] 1.96, 95% CI 1.15 to 3.33) and reduced the need for oral antibiotics (3 studies, n = 527; OR 0.28, 95% CI 0.19 to 0.42) [56]. In a double-blind, randomised, controlled trial for CF patients aged 6–18 years the serum markers of inflammation (myeloperoxidase, high-sensitivity C-reactive protein, intracellular adhesion molecule 1, IL-6, calprotectin, serum amyloid A and G-CSF) showed significant reduction at the 6-month evaluation in the treated group compared to non-treated one [84].

Based on this extensive knowledge for the benefits to patients with CF, the CF Foundation recommends the chronic administration of azithromycin to all CF patients aged six years and older who are infected with *P. aeruginosa*. Nevertheless, this therapy could be considered in those patients who are not infected with *P. aeruginosa*, too [85]. A similar recommendation is noted in the NICE guidelines [86].

Regarding the posology and duration of treatment, Wilms and colleagues demonstrated that a dose of 22–30 mg/kg/week was the lowest with validated therapeutic efficacy, where the weekly dose can be divided into 1–7 administrations, depending on patient preference and gastrointestinal tolerance [87]. However, the positive effects have been seen for the first year, and afterward, there is a steady level of lung function with not improve further on. Therefore, it was concluded that azithromycin therapy should be limited to 6–12 months because, after this period, the risk of adverse reactions and other drug-related problems could outweigh the benefits [88].

CONCLUSION

The inflammatory response to lung infection in CF patients is ineffective; moreover, the immune responses lead to severe and persistent consequences. Thus, high-intensity inflammation that does not resolve induces permanent damage of the airways, impairs lung function and, if undiagnosed, eventually causes respiratory failure and death. Functional CFTR is essential to ensure that the pathogen-associated airway inflammation is adequate.

Therefore the future belongs to CFTR modulators that hopefully could provide functionality of CFTR in all patients until then any possible therapeutical interaction into the inflammatory cascade is crucial to clear pathogens and preserve normal tissue function. A more in-depth understanding of the IL-17-related pathways in the context of CF lung disease is critical to assess the potential implications of anti-IL-17 therapy or interventions targeting its cellular source.

REFERENCES

[1] Smyth, AR; Bell, SC; Bojcin, S; et al. European Cystic Fibrosis Society Standards of Care Best Practice guidelines. *J Cyst Fibros*, 2014, 13(1), S23–S42.

[2] Simmonds, NJ; Cullinan, P; Hodson, ME. Growing old with cystic fibrosis—the characteristics of long-term survivors of cystic fibrosis. *Respir Med*, 2009, 103, 29–35.

[3] O'Sullivan, BP; Freedman, SD. Cystic fibrosis. *Lancet*, 2009, 373, 1891–1904.

[4] Rossi, GA; Morelli, P; Galietta, LJ; Colin, AA. Airway microenvironment alterations and pathogen growth in cystic fibrosis. *Pediatric Pulmonology*, 2019, 54, 497– 506.

[5] Stoltz, DA; Meyerholz, DK; Welsh, MJ. Origins of cystic fibrosis lung disease. *N Engl J Med.*, 2015, 372, 351-62.

[6] Khan, TZ; Wagener, JS; Bost, T; Martinez, J; Accurso, FJ; Riches, DW. Early pulmonary inflammation in infants with cystic fibrosis. *Am J Respir Crit Care Med.*, 1995, 151, 1075-82.

[7] Stick, S; Tiddens, H; Aurora, P; Gustafsson, P; Ranganathan, S; Robinson, P; Rosenfeld, M; Sly, P; Ratjen, F. Early intervention studies in infants and preschool children with cystic fibrosis: are we ready? *Eur Respir J.*, 2013, 42, 527-38.

[8] Ramsey, KA; Ranganathan, S; Park, J; Skoric, B; Adams, AM; Simpson, SJ; Robins-Browne, RM; Franklin, PJ; de Klerk, NH; Sly, PD; et al. Early respiratory infection is associated with reduced spirometry in children with cystic fibrosis. *Am J Respir Crit Care Med*, 2014, 190, 1111-6.

[9] Mott, LS; Park, J; Murray, CP; Gangell, CL; de Klerk, NH; Robinson, PJ; Robertson, CF; Ranganathan, SC; Sly, PD; Stick, SM; et al. Progression of early structural lung disease in young children with cystic fibrosis assessed using CT. *Thorax*, 2012, 67, 509-16.

[10] Tang, AC; Turvey, SE; Alves, MP; Regamey, N; Tümmler, B; Hartl, D. Current concepts: host-pathogen interactions in cystic fibrosis airways disease. *Eur Respir Rev*, 2014, 23, 320-32.

[11] Furukawa, BS; Flume, PA. Nontuberculous Mycobacteria in Cystic Fibrosis, *Semin Respir Crit Care Med*, 2018, 39(03), 383-39, 1. Cohen-Cymberknoh, M; Kerem, E; Ferkol, T; Elizur, A. Airway inflammation in cystic fibrosis: molecular mechanisms and clinical implications. *Thorax*, 2013, 68, 1157-62.

[12] Fahy, JV; Dickey, BF. Airway mucus function and dysfunction. *N Engl J Med*, 2010, 363, 2233-47.

[13] Lovewell, RR; Patankar, YR; Berwin, B. Mechanisms of phagocytosis and host clearance of Pseudomonas aeruginosa. *Am J Physiol Lung Cell Mol Physiol*, 2014, 306, L591-603.

[14] Nichols, DP; Chmiel, JF. Inflammation and its genesis in cystic fibrosis. *Pediatric Pulmonology*, 2015, 50, S39–S56.

[15] Davies, JC. Pseudomonas aeruginosa in cystic fibrosis: pathogenesis and persistence. *Pediatr. Respir. Rev*, 2003, 3, 128-134.

[16] Mauch, RM; Levy, CE. Serum antibodies to Pseudomonas aeruginosa in cystic fibrosis: a systematic review. *J Cyst Fibros*, 2014, 13(5), 499–507.

[17] Doring, G. Host response to Pseudomonas aeruginosa. *Acta Paediatr Scand*, 1989, Suppl 363, 37–39.

[18] Markham, RB; Powderly, WG. Exposure of mice to live Pseudomonas aeruginosa generates protective cell-mediated immunity in the absence of an antibody response. *J Immunol*, 1988, 140, 2039–2045.

[19] Marvig, RL; Sommer, LM; Molin, S; Johansen, HK. Convergent evolution and adaptation of Pseudomonas aeruginosa within patients with cystic fibrosis. *Nature Genetics*, 2015, 47, 57-54.

[20] Strateva, T; Yordanov, D. Pseudomonas aeruginosa - a phenomenon of bacterial resistance. *J Med Microbiol*, 2009, 58(9), 1133-48.

[21] Strateva, T; Petrova, G; Perenovska, P; Mitov, I. Bulgarian cystic fibrosis Pseudomonas aeruginosa isolates: antimicrobial susceptibility and neuraminidase-encoding gene distribution *J Med Microbiol*, 2009, 58(5), 690-2.

[22] Esther, CR; Jr. Lin, FC; Kerr, A; Miller, MB; Gilligan, PH. Respiratory viruses are associated with common respiratory pathogens in cystic fibrosis. *Pediatr Pulmonol*, 2014, 49, 926-31.

[23] Hartl, D; Griese, M; Kappler, M; Zissel, G; Reinhardt, D; Rebhan, C; et al. Pulmonary T(H)2 response in Pseudomonas aeruginosa-infected patients with cystic fibrosis. *J Allergy Clin Immunol*, 2006, 117, 204–211.8.

[24] Tang, XX; Fok, KL; Chen, H; Chan, KS; Tsang, LL; Rowlands, DK; et al. Lymphocyte CFTR promotes epithelial bicarbonate secretion for bacterial killing. *J Cell Physiol.*, 2012, 227, 3887–3894.

[25] Mulcahy, EM; Hudson, JB; Beggs, SA; Reid, DW; Roddam, LF; Cooley, MA. High Peripheral Blood Th17 Percent Associated with Poor Lung Function in Cystic Fibrosis. *PLoS ONE*, 2015, 10(3), e0120912.

[26] Mueller, C; Braag, SA; Keeler, A; Hodges, C; Drumm, M; Flotte, TR. Lack of cystic fibrosis transmembrane conductance regulator in

CD3+ lymphocytes leads to aberrant cytokine secretion and hyperinflammatory adaptive immune responses. *Am J Respir Cell Mol Biol*, 2011, 44, 922–929.

[27] Moss, RB. Pathophysiology and immunology of allergic bronchopulmonary aspergillosis. *Med Mycol*, 2005, 43 Suppl 1, S203-6.,

[28] Knutsen, AP; Slavin, RG. Allergic bronchopulmonary aspergillosis in asthma and cystic fibrosis. *Clin Dev Immunol.*, 2011, 843763.

[29] Lutzky, VP; Ratnatunga, CN; Smith, DJ; et al. Anomalies in T Cell Function Are Associated With Individuals at Risk of Mycobacterium abscessus Complex Infection. *Front Immunol*, 2018, 9, 1319.

[30] Chan, YR; Chen, K; Duncan, SR; Lathrop, KL; Latoche, JD; Logar, AJ; et al. Patients with cystic fibrosis have inducible IL-17+IL-22+ memory cells in lung draining lymph nodes. *J Allergy Clin Immunol*, 2013, 131, 1117–1129, 1129 e1111–1115.

[31] Anil, N; Singh, M. CD4(+)CD25(high) FOXP3(+) regulatory T cells correlate with FEV1 in North Indian children with cystic fibrosis. *Immunol Invest*, 2013, 43, 535–543.

[32] Bernardi, DM; Ribeiro, AF; Mazzola, TN; Vilela, MM; Sgarbieri, VC. The impact of cystic fibrosis on the immunologic profile of pediatric patients. *J Pediatr (Rio J).*, 2013, 89, 40–47.

[33] Smith, DJ; Hill, GR; Bell, SC; Reid, DW. Reduced mucosal associated invariant T-cells are associated with increased disease severity and Pseudomonas aeruginosa infection in cystic fibrosis. *PLoS One*, 2014, 9, e109891.

[34] Regamey, N; Tsartsali, L; Hilliard, TN; Fuchs, O; Tan, HL; Zhu, J; Qiu, YS; Alton, EW; Jeffery, PK; Bush, A; et al. Distinct patterns of inflammation in the airway lumen and bronchial mucosa of children with cystic fibrosis. *Thorax*, 2012, 67, 164–170.

[35] Tan, Hui-leng. The Th17 pathway in Cystic Fibrosis lung disease, research thesis for medical degree, *National Heart & Lung Institute Imperial College*, London, 2011.

[36] Tiringer, K; Treis, A; Fucik, P; Gona, M; Gruber, S; Renner, S; et al. A Th17- and Th2-skewed cytokine profile in cystic fibrosis lungs

represents a potential risk factor for Pseudomonas aeruginosa infection. *Am J Respir Crit Care Med.*, 2013, 187, 621–629.

[37] Henry, RL; Mellis, CM; Petrovic, L. *Mucoid Pseudomonas aeruginosa is a marker of poor survival in cystic fibrosis Pediatric Pulmonology*, 1992, 12, 158-161.

[38] Emerson, J; Rosenfeld, M; McNamara, S; Ramsey, B; Gibson, R. Pseudomonas aeruginosa and other predictors of mortality and morbidity in young children with cystic fibrosis. *Pediatr Pulmonol*, 2005, 34, 91–100.

[39] Dubin, PJ; McAllister, F; Kolls, JK. Is cystic fibrosis a TH17 disease? *Inflamm Res.*, 2007, 56, 221-7.

[40] Newcomb, DC; Peebles, RS. Jr. Th17-mediated inflammation in asthma. *Curr Opin Immunol.*, 2013, 25, 755-60.

[41] Lee, RJ; Foskett, JK. Ca(2)(+) signaling and fluid secretion by secretory cells of the airway epithelium. *Cell Calcium.*, 2014, 55, 325–336.

[42] McLoughlin, RM; Calatroni, A; Visness, CM; Wallace, PK; Cruikshank, WW; Tuzoava, M; et al. Longitudinal relationship of early life immunomodulatory T cell phenotype and function to development of allergic sensitization in an urban cohort. *Clin Exp Allergy.*, 2012, 42, 392–404.

[43] Holt, PG. Infection and the development of allergic disease. *Allergy.*, 2011, 66, Suppl 95, 13–15.

[44] Velikova, T; et al. Th17 cells in Bulgarian children with chronic obstructive lung diseases. *Allergol Immunopathol (Madr).*, 2019, 47(3), 227-233.

[45] Iannitti, RG; Carvalho, A; Cunha, C; De Luca, A; Giovannini, G; Casagrande, A; Zelante, T; Vacca, C; Fallarino, F; Puccetti, P; et al. Th17/Treg imbalance in murine cystic fibrosis is linked to indoleamine 2,3-dioxygenase deficiency but corrected by kynurenines. *Am J Respir Crit Care Med*, 2013, 187, 609–620.

[46] Robinson, KM; Alcorn, JF. T-cell immunotherapy in cystic fibrosis: weighing the risk/reward. *Am J Respir Crit Care Med*, 2013, 187, 564–566.

[47] Parfenova, EN; Ryviakova, EV. [Use of erythromycin in non-specific inflammatory diseases of the Urogenital System]. *Urol Mosc*, 1963, 28, 29–31.

[48] Plewig, G; Schopf, E. Anti-inflammatory effects of antimicrobial agents: an *in vivo* study. *J Invest Dermatol*, 1975, 65(6), 532–6.

[49] Zuckerman, JM. Macrolides and ketolides, azithromycin; clarithromycin, telithromycin. *Infect Dis Clin North Am*, 2004, 18(3), 621–49.

[50] Kudoh, S; Azuma, A; Yamamoto, M; Izumi, T; Ando, M. Improvement of survival in patients with diffuse panbronchiolitis treated with low-dose erythromycin. *Am J Respir Crit Care Med*, 1998, 157(6 Pt 1), 1829–32.

[51] Koutsoubari, I; Papaevangelou, V; Konstantinou, GN; Makrinioti, H; Xepapadaki, P; Kafetzis, D; et al. Effect of clarithromycin on acute asthma exacerbations in children: an open randomized study. *Pediatr Allergy Immunol*, 2012, 23(4), 385–90.

[52] Clement, A; Tamalet, A; Leroux, E; Ravilly, S; Fauroux, B; Jais, JP. Long term effects of azithromycin in patients with cystic fibrosis: a double blind; placebo controlled trial. *Thorax*, 2006, 61(10), 895–902.

[53] Wong, C; Jayaram, L; Karalus, N; Eaton, T; Tong, C; Hockey, H; et al. Azithromycin for prevention of exacerbations in non-cystic fibrosis bronchiectasis (EMBRACE): a randomised, double-blind, placebo-controlled trial. *Lancet*, 2012, 380(9842), 660–7.

[54] Donath, E; Chaudhry, A; Hernandez-Aya, LF; Lit, L. A meta-analysis on the prophylactic use of macrolide antibiotics for the prevention of disease exacerbations in patients with Chronic Obstructive Pulmonary Disease. *Respir Med*, 2013, 107(9), 1385–92.

[55] Southern, KW; Barker, PM; Solis-Moya, A; Patel, L. Macrolide antibiotics for cystic fibrosis. *Cochrane Database Syst Rev*, 2012, 11, Cd002203.

[56] Rodvold, KA. Clinical pharmacokinetics of clarithromycin. *Clin Pharmacokinet*, 1999, 37(5), 385–98.

[57] Foulds, G; Shepard, RM; Johnson, RB. The pharmacokinetics of azithromycin in human serum and tissues. *J Antimicrob Chemother*, 1990, 25, (Suppl A), 73–82.

[58] Dette, GA. [Tissue penetration of erythromycin]. *Infection*, 1979, 7(3), 129–45.

[59] Parnham, MJ. Immunomodulatory effects of antimicrobials in the therapy of respiratory tract infections. *Curr Opin Infect Dis*, 2015, 18, 125–131.

[60] Zimmermann, P; Ziesenitz, VC; Curtis, N; Ritz, N. The Immunomodulatory Effects of Macrolides—A Systematic Review of the Underlying Mechanisms. *Front. Immunol.*, 2018, 9, 302.

[61] Bosnar, M; Čužić, S; Bošnjak, B; Nujić, K; Ergović, G; Marjanović, N; et al. Azithromycin inhibits macrophage interleukin-1beta production through inhibition of activator protein-1 in lipopolysaccharide-induced murine pulmonary neutrophilia. *Int Immunopharmacol*, 2011, 11(4), 424–34.

[62] Cheung, PS; Si, EC; Hosseini, K. Anti-inflammatory activity of azithromycin as measured by its NF-kappaB, inhibitory activity. *Ocul Immunol Inflamm*, 2010, 18(1), 32–7.

[63] Cigana, C; Nicolis, E; Pasetto, M; Assael, BM; Melotti, P. Anti-inflammatory effects of azithromycin in cystic fibrosis airway epithelial cells. *Biochem Biophys Res Commun*, 2006, 350(4), 977–82.

[64] Park, SJ; Lee, YC; Rhee, YK; Lee, HB. The effect of long-term treatment with erythromycin on Th1 and Th2 cytokines in diffuse panbronchiolitis. *Biochem Biophys Res Commun*, 2004, 324(1), 114–7.

[65] Kobayashi, M; Shimauchi, T; Hino, R; Tokura, Y. Roxithromycin downmodulates Th2 chemokine production by keratinocytes and chemokine receptor expression on Th2 cells: its dual inhibitory effects on the ligands and the receptors. *Cell Immunol*, 2004, 228(1), 27–33.

[66] Ivetić Tkalčević, V; Cužić, S; Kramarić, MD; Parnham, MJ; Eraković Haber, V. Topical azithromycin and clarithromycin inhibit

acute and chronic skin inflammation in sensitized mice, with apparent selectivity for Th2-mediated processes in delayed-type hypersensitivity. *Inflammation*, 2012, 35(1), 192– 205.

[67] Marjanović, N; Bosnar, M; Michielin, F; Willé, DR; Anić-Milić, T; Culić, O; et al. Macrolide antibiotics broadly and distinctively inhibit cytokine and chemokine production by COPD sputum cells *in vitro*. *Pharmacol Res*, 2011, 63, 389–397.

[68] Hodge, S; Hodge, G; Jersmann, H; Matthews, G; Ahern, J; Holmes, M; et al. Azithromycin improves macrophage phagocytic function and expression of mannose receptor in chronic obstructive pulmonary disease. *Am J Respir Crit Care Med*, 2008, 178, 139–148.

[69] Yamauchi, K; Shibata, Y; Kimura, T; Abe, S; Inoue, S; Osaka, D; et al. Azithromycin suppresses interleukin-12p40 expression in lipopolysaccharide and interferon-gamma stimulatedmacrophages. *Int J Biol Sci*, 2009, 23, 667–678.

[70] Ito, T; Ito, N; Hashizume, H; Takigawa, M. Roxithromycin inhibits chemokine-induced chemotaxis of Th1 and Th2 cells but regulatory T cells. *J Dermatol Sci*, 2009, 54(3), 185–91.

[71] Gualdoni, GA; Lingscheid, T; Schmetterer, KG; Hennig, A; Steinberger, P; Zlabinger, GJ. Azithromycin inhibits IL-1 secretion and non-canonical inflammasome activation. *Sci Rep*, 2015, 5, 12016.

[72] Sato, Y; Kaneko, K; Inoue, M. Macrolide antibiotics promote the LPS-induced upregulation of prostaglandin E receptor EP2 and thus attenuate macrolide suppression of IL-6 production. *Prostaglandins Leukot Essent Fatty Acids*, 2007, 76(3), 181–8.

[73] Wuyts, WA; Willems, S; Vos, R; et al. Azithromycin reduces pulmonary fibrosis in a bleomycin mouse model, *Experimental Lung Research*, 2010, 36, 10, 602-614.

[74] Linden, A; Laan, M; Anderson, GP. Neutrophils, interleukin-17A and lung disease. *Eur Respir J.*, 2005, 25, 159–172.

[75] Vanaudenaerde, BM; De Vleeschauwer, SI; Vos, R; et al. The role of the IL23/IL17 axis in bronchiolitis obliterans syndrome after lung transplantation. *Am J Transplant.*, 2008, 8, 1911–1920.

[76] Parnham, MJ; Erakovic Haber, V; Giamarellos-Bourboulis, EJ; Perletti, G; Verleden, GM; Vos, R. Azithromycin: mechanisms of action and their relevance for clinical applications. *Pharmacol Ther*, 2014, 143, 225–245.

[77] Halldorsson, S; Gudjonsson, T; Gottfredsson, M; Singh, PK; Gudmundsson, GH; Baldursson, O. Azithromycin maintains airway epithelial integrity during Pseudomonas aeruginosa infection. *Am J Respir Cell Mol Biol*, 2010, 42, 62–680.

[78] Imamura, Y; Yanagihara, K; Mizuta, Y; Seki, M; Ohno, H; Higashiyama, Y; et al. Azithromycin inhibits MUC5AC production induced by the Pseudomonas aeruginosa autoinducer N-(3-Oxododecanoyl) homoserine lactone in NCI-H292 Cells. *Antimicrob Agents Chemother*, 2014, 48, 3457–3461.

[79] Daenas, C; Hatziefthimiou, AA; Gourgoulianis, KI; Molyvdas, PA. Azithromycin has a direct relaxant effect on precontracted airway smooth muscle. *Eur J Pharmacol*, 2006, 553, 280–287.

[80] Willems-Widyastuti, A; Vanaudenaerde, BM; Vos, R; Dilisen, E; Verleden, SE; De Vleeschauwer, SI; et al. Azithromycin attenuates fibroblast growth factors induced vascular endothelial growth factor via p38(MAPK) signaling in human airway smooth muscle cells. *Cell Biochem Biophys*, 2013, 67, 331–339.

[81] Saiman, L; Anstead, M; Mayer-Hamblett, N; Lands, LC; Kloster, M; Hocevar-Trnka, J; et al. Effect of azithromycin on pulmonary function in patients with cystic fibrosis uninfected with Pseudomonas aeruginosa: a randomized controlled trial. *JAMA*, 2010, 303, 1707–15.

[82] Saiman, L; Mayer-Hamblett, N; Anstead, M; Lands, LC; Kloster, M; Goss, CH; et al. Open-label, follow-on study of azithromycin in pediatric patients with CF uninfected with Pseudomonas aeruginosa. *Pediatr Pulmonol*, 2012, 47, 641–8.

[83] Ratjen, F; Saiman, L; Mayer-Hamblett, N; Lands, LC; Kloster, M; Thompson, V; et al. Effect of azithromycin on systemic markers of inflammation in patients with cystic fibrosis uninfected with Pseudomonas aeruginosa. *Chest*, 2012, 142, 1259–1266.

[84] Mogayzel, Jr. PJ; Naureckas, ET; Robinson, KA; Mueller, G; Hadjiliadis, D; Hoag, JB; et al. Cystic fibrosis pulmonary guidelines. Chronic medications for maintenance of lung health. *Am J Respir Crit Care Med*, 2013, 187, 680–9).

[85] Cystic fifibrosis: long-term azithromycin (ESUOM37) Evidence summary, Published, 25 November 2014, last access at https://www.nice.org.uk/advice/esuom37/chapter/full-evidence-summary on 28.10.2019.

[86] Wilms, EB; Touw, DJ; Heijerman, HG; van der Ent, CK. Azithromycin maintenance therapy in patients with cystic fibrosis: a dose advice based on a review of pharmacokinetics, efficacy, and side effects. *Pediatr Pulmonol*, 2012, 47, 658–665.

[87] Willekens, J; Eyns, H; Malfroot, A. How long should we maintain long-term azithromycin treatment in cystic fibrosis patients? *Pediatr Pulmonol*, 2015, 50, 103–104.

In: Th17 Cells in Health and Disease
ISBN: 978-1-53617-152-5
Editor: Tsvetelina Velikova
© 2020 Nova Science Publishers, Inc.

Chapter 8

MULTIPLE SCLEROSIS: TH17 CELLS IN IMMUNOPATHOGENESIS AND THERAPY

Marina Ivanova[1,*], MD, Ivan Milanov[1], MD, PhD,
Ekaterina Krasimirova[2], MD, PhD,
Dobroslav Kyurkchiev[2], MD, PhD
and Tsvetelina Velikova[3], MD, PhD

[1]Clinic of Neurology, University Hospital of Neurology
and Psychiatry "St. Naum," Sofia, Bulgaria
Department of Neurology, Faculty of Medicine,
Medical University of Sofia, Sofia, Bulgaria
[2]Laboratory of Clinical Immunology, University Hospital
"St. Ivan Rilski," Department of Clinical Immunology,
Medical Faculty, Medical University of Sofia, Sofia, Bulgaria
[3]Clinical Immunology, University Hospital Lozenetz,
Sofia University, Sofia, Bulgaria

---

* Corresponding Author's Email: marinaivanova1900@gmail.com.

ABSTRACT

Multiple sclerosis (MS) is a chronic autoimmune disease of the central nervous system with neurodegenerative and inflammatory features and still unrevealed etiology. The prevalence of MS worldwide remains high.

Th17 cells are involved in the pathogenesis of MS confirmed by an experimental model of autoimmune encephalomyelitis. Due to pathogenic processes in CNS and disrupted the blood-brain barrier, Th17 cells and their respective cytokines act locally and distal via the peripheral blood. IL-17, IL-6, TNFα, and IL-22 contribute to inflammatory and demyelination process of the neurons, therefore add to the clinical picture.

Knowing the causes of resistance to therapy of some MS patients would benefit the development and improvement of immunomodulatory treatment for the disease. There is still no clarity on why the treatment stops being effective and the disease progresses. Searching for new markers for predicting the risk of attacks or disease worsening and for monitoring the effect of immunomodulatory therapy in MS patients continues.

Keywords: multiple sclerosis, Th17 cells, IL-17, immunomodulatory therapy

INTRODUCTION

Multiple sclerosis (MS) remains the most common chronic inflammatory and demyelinating disease of the central nervous system (CNS) [1]. The condition has a chronic course and affects mainly young people between the ages of 20 and 40 years [2]. MS is the second major cause of motor disability in young and middle-aged people [3], with more than 2.5 million people suffering from the disease worldwide [2].

The symptoms of the disease are due to two major pathological processes - focal inflammation and neurodegeneration. Inflammation leads to segmental demyelination of the white matter with plaque formation and axonal degeneration and neuronal damage [4]. Chronic fatigue syndrome, depression, and cognitive impairment are common symptoms that disrupt daily activities and contribute to the disability of patients [5-7].

MULTIPLE SCLEROSIS AS AN AUTOIMMUNE DISEASE

MS is an example of an autoimmune disease where impaired tolerance to own tissues has been described, with a subsequent pathological immune attack against individual cells and tissues [4].

The condition is also classified in the group of demyelinating inflammatory diseases and neurodegenerative diseases [2, 4, 5, 8]. MS damages the myelin sheath of the nerve fibers in the CNS. The relation between neurodegeneration and demyelination in the pathophysiology of MS is a matter of debate, especially knowing that some MS lesions occur in the absence of inflammation.

Some authors suggest the involvement of activated microglia and oligodendrocytes in the absence of inflammation as the cause of CNS damage [1]. However, there are various immune mechanisms involved in the pathogenesis of MS lesions that have not been fully understood.

The disease etiology remains unknown [3]. MS development is thought to be the result of an abnormal response of the immune system to one or more myelin sheath antigens, developing this reaction in genetically predisposed individuals [9]. The impact of various causes such as genetic factors, gender, racial differences, viruses, lifestyle, and deficiency of vitamins, antioxidants, probiotics, and nutrients in food is also discussed. Viral infections, such as herpes viruses, Epstein - Barr virus, varicella-zoster virus, HHV 6, are considered as an etiological factor but remain unproven [3].

Recently, there was the dilemma of whether MS is a primary CNS degenerative disease with secondary onset inflammation, or is an autoimmune disease with the development of immune-mediated CNS lesion. However, allelic variants in MS and other autoimmune disorders in the Genome-wide association study (GWAS) provides reliable data on the autoimmune genesis of MS [5].

ROLE OF TH17 CELLS IN THE PATHOGENESIS OF MULTIPLE SCLEROSIS

Much of the knowledge about the immunopathogenesis of the disease is explained by the model of experimental autoimmune encephalomyelitis (EAE). In EAE, animals (most often rats and mice) are immunized with different myelin proteins, i.e., myelin basic protein (BPM), myelin periphery protein (MPP), and myelin oligodendrocyte glycoprotein (MOG) [3, 6]. EAE can also be induced in non-immunized animals by transferring specific activated T cells that recognize myelin antigens [3].

EAE model represents the induction of MS symptoms by autoreactive T cells (CD4+) attacking antigens in CNS myelin [2]. A complex cascade of events occurs associated with the release of proinflammatory cytokines, expression of adhesive molecules and secretion of matrix metalloproteinases, with disruption of the blood-brain barrier and additional invasion of activated T cells in the CNS [1].

Several types of T helper cells are described: Th1, Th2, Th9, Th17, Th22 [5, 6]. Pathogenesis in MS is associated with the complex involvement of CD8+ T cytotoxic cells, macrophages, NK cells, and microglia as well [2]. Th1 cells that are activated by endogenous peptides presented with MHC class I lead to the secretion of IFNγ, IL-2, TNFα, and are defined as proinflammatory cells in the mechanism of EAE [5]. By cytokines that produce, they activate macrophages, cellular immunity, and secretion of antibodies by B cells. Th2 lymphocytes mainly produce IL-4, IL-5, IL-10, and IL-13, which promote humoral immunity but can act as anti-inflammatory factors that may have a protective role for EAE. Based on the previously mentioned findings, Th1/Th17 conception replaces the classical Th1 paradigm in both EAE and MS. It was postulated that Th17 cells would play a more critical role in the initial phases of EAE and MS, whileTh1 cells would be more important in later stages of the inflammation in the CNS [10].

As described above, T-helper cells play an essential role in the initiation of MS and the progression of the disease. In MS, the

Multiple Sclerosis

inflammatory process is mediated mainly by IL-17 and IFNγ. It was demonstrated that IL-17 represents a family of cytokines, which includes IL-17A to IL-17F [10]. The increased amount of Th17 cells, especially in the area of active brain lesions, is associated with the severity of the disease.

The differentiation of CD4+ naïve T cells into Th17 cells is mediated by IL-21 and IL-23 and potently inhibited by IFN-γ and IL-4 [10]. IL-23 is produced by antigen-presenting cells, e.g., dendritic cells and macrophages that are "loaded" with antigens that activate autoreactive Th17 cells. Therefore, Th17 cells are mainly found in the inflammatory areas of the CNS and can be identified with the expression of the IL-23R receptor. However, the differentiation of T naive cells intoTh17 cells may be maintained not only by IL-23 but also by the combination of TGF-β1 and IL-6. A significant proportion of IL-17-producing (i.e., Th17) cells may convert into IFN-γ-producing T cells. It is assumed that this happens due to IL-23-mediated reprogramming [14]. There is also a subset of cells that simultaneously express IFN-γ and have chemokine receptors from both Th17 and Th1 cells [10].

Th17 cells are thought to be more pro-inflammatory cells. They secrete IL-17A, IL-17 F, IL-21, and IL-22, which are associated with the onset of various autoimmune diseases [5, 11, 12]. In line with this, there is evidence that IL-17 presents in high concentrations in the blood and the CNS in MS patients, particularly during exacerbations of the disease. *In vitro* studies demonstrated that the IL-17, along with IL-5, were produced by mononuclear cells obtained from patients with MS in cultures after stimulation with human myelin basic protein. The level of IL-17 was shown to correlate with the number of active lesions on magnetic resonance imaging (MRI). The proportion of Th17 cells and their memory counterpart (CD4+/CD45RO+/CCR7−), together with the level of IL-17A correlated with disease activity, evaluated by the Expanded Disability Status Scale (EDSS). However, the central memory Th17 cells (CD4+/CD45RO+/CCR7+) were associated with relapse frequency. Besides, serum IL-17F (but not IL-17A) correlated with the number of MS relapses in two years [10].

Increased numbers of IL-17- producing T cells are detected in MS and EAE lesions. It was found that IL-17 itself can not initiate EAE, but is an essential factor in neuroinflammation. IL-17 contributes to the severity of MS by stimulating the secretion of IL-6 of microglia and astrocytes.

As a result, the accumulated neutrophils deteriorate endothelial dysfunction through the destruction of proteins that bind endothelial cells. IL-17 acts synergistically with TNF-α by stimulating the production of E-selectin, P-selectin, GM-CSF, and G-CSF by endothelial and other epithelial cells, which lead to uncontrolled oxidative stress and death of oligodendrocytes [12].

Th22 cells are the primary sources of IL-22 and exert a vital role in the pathogenesis of MS by producing chemokines and disruption of the blood-brain barrier. In contrast to Th17 cells, which increase during MS onset, an increased percentage of Th22 cells in peripheral blood are detected one month before exacerbation of the disease [13]. It could be speculated that these cells are involved in the initiation of relapses by communicating with autoreactive T cells that have crossed the blood-brain barrier [13], but more research is needed to clarify these mechanisms.

TNFα is one of the major pro-inflammatory cytokines found in high blood concentrations in patients with MS. It is produced by macrophages, microglia, and CD 4+ T cells. Together with INFγ and IL-17, it stimulates the synthesis of chemokines and adhesion molecules by endothelial cells and contributes to the disruption of the blood-brain barrier. TNFα is also detected in the demyelinating regions of the CNS and has been shown to lead to the death of oligodendrocytes [12].

In local lymph nodes, autoreactive Th1 cells recognize the antigens represented by macrophages and dendritic cells, activate and secrete pro-inflammatory cytokines [4]. To reach the site of inflammation, Th1 lymphocytes must move to cross the blood-brain barrier. This is accomplished through chemokines and various adhesion molecules that support trans-endothelial migration [3] via diapedesis [14]. Th17 cells are also involved in the process by secretion of IL-17. This violates the integrity of the blood-brain barrier, leading to an infiltration of Th1, CD8+ cytotoxic cells, B lymphocytes, etc. [3]. It is thought that an increased percentage of Th17 cells and secretion of their respective cytokines could be correlated with the risk of relapse or worsening of the disease symptoms.

When entering into the brain, autoreactive T cells attack the corresponding antigen. These antigens are not naïve but presented on the surface of antigen-presenting cells, such as macrophages, microglial, and astroglial cells [3, 14]. Through INFγ and TNFα, T cells induce macrophages that destroy oligodendrocytes and myelin [3]. In addition to the mechanisms of the cell-mediated immune response, humoral mechanisms are also involved. On the one hand, autoreactive T cells trigger the immune response, including activation of innate immunity (i.e., complement) that directly damages oligodendrocytes [3] and, on the other hand, B lymphocytes produce autoreactive antibodies [4].

The characteristic neuropathological substrate of MS is the formation of a plaque of demyelination with reactive gliosis around it [14]. Most plaques are located around a central vein that has a damaged and permeable blood-brain barrier [3]. Immunohistological analysis has revealed that the plaque contains deposits of antibodies, autoreactive T cells, macrophages, antigens, adhesion molecules, chemokines, and cytokines [14]. T cells and macrophages or activated microglia [3] are dominant in plaque. In the final stage of demyelination, macrophages phagocytize the myelin sheaths, which leads to axonal damage and disturbance in the normal conduction of nerve impulses [3, 4].

Some authors determine differences in the immunological status among different MS clinical subtypes. Arellano et al. collect blood samples from untreated patients diagnosed with clinically isolated syndrome, various clinical forms of MS and healthy controls. The samples were tested for plasma levels of interferon (IFN)-γ, IL-10, TGF-β, IL-17A, and IL-17F, Th1, and Th17 cells in the periphery. Th1 cells were found more abundant in clinically isolated syndrome and relapsing-remitting MS than in progressive MS, and relapsing-remitting MS had a higher percentage of Th17 cells than the clinically isolated syndrome. Moreover, the Th1/Th17 cell ratio was skewed toward Th1 in clinically isolated syndrome compared to MS phenotypes and healthy controls. Interestingly, relapsing-remitting

MS patients had a significantly higher Th1 cell frequency than secondary progressive MS and primary progressive MS patients [15].

In contrast, the number of Th17 cells was lower in clinically isolated syndrome patients than in relapsing-remitting MS patients. Remarkably, clinically isolated syndrome patients had a significantly higher Th1/Th17 ratio than healthy subjects and relapsing-remitting MS, secondary progressive MS, and primary-porgressive MS patients. In line with this, the Th1/Th17 cell ratio, together with the IFN-γ/IL-17F cytokine ratio indicates the progression from a Th1 phenotype toward a Th17 phenotype as disease evolves from clinically isolated syndrome to relapsing-remitting MS or primary progressive subtypes. They found that clinically isolated syndrome patients had a lower Th17 cell frequency than relapsing-remitting MS [15].

Th17 cells are considered as vital regulators of disease severity in MS. However, Th17 cells are functionally heterogeneous, consisting of subpopulations that differentially may produce IL-17, IFNγ, and granulocyte-macrophage colony-stimulating factor (GM-SCF), mostly depending on the species and pro-inflammatory milieu. Langelaar et al. examined the different effector phenotypes of human Th17 cells and their correlation with disease activity in MS patients [16].

They found low frequencies of Th1-like Th17 (CCR6+CXCR3+), but not Th17 (CCR6+CXCR3-) effector memory populations in blood. Moreover, these cells were strongly associated with clinically definite MS. In MS patients with clinically isolated syndrome and relapsing-remitting form, Th1-like Th17 effector memory cells were abundant in the cerebrospinal fluid and showed increased production of IFNγ and GM-CSF compared to paired CCR6+ and CCR6-CD8+ T cell populations and their blood equivalents after short-term culturing. Therefore, the potential of Th17 cells to infiltrate the central nervous system was supported by their predominance in the cerebrospinal fluid of early MS patients. These findings spread light on the dominant contribution of Th1-like Th17 lymphocytes, in particular Th17 cells, to clinical disease activity. They demonstrated that IFNγ- and GM-CSF-expressing Th1-like Th17 cells are selectively associated with early disease activity in patients with MS [16].

IMMUNOMODULATORY THERAPY WITH BETA-INTERFERON DRUGS AND FINGOLIMOD

Several studies have been conducted worldwide to identify reliable markers (clinical and biological) to monitor the effect of immunomodulatory therapy in patients with MS. Due to the role of Th17 lymphocytes in the pathogenesis of the disease, more studies are being undertaken to evaluate the therapeutic response to treatment, especially with biological therapies such as beta-interferons and fingolimod. For example, when detecting patients' percentages of Th17 lymphocytes and levels of their respective cytokines close to the levels in healthy controls, and in the absence of clinical deterioration, it could be argued that we have an excellent response to therapy. In the case of increased levels of investigated immunological markers and clinical deterioration, it is possible to assume that the patients are resistant to the treatment and do not respond well to treatment.

Esendagli et al. described 15 patients with relapsing MS, eight patients with progressive MS, and eight healthy controls. They examined the levels of IL-17, IL-23, IL-26, and IL-17R before initiating beta-interferon therapy and two years after treatment. Patients with progressive MS were monitored before starting immunosuppressants [17]. In their study also observed high levels of IL-17 and IL-17R in patients with progressive MS and nonresponsive patients. Additionally, IL-23 and IL-26 levels were increased, suggesting that this is most likely due to compensatory mechanisms to maintain IL-17 levels low during beta-interferon treatment.

The authors found that IL-17 and IL-17R receptor levels significantly decreased during the 2-year beta-interferon treatment in responders to the therapy. Therefore, measurement of the IL-17 and IL-17R receptor may be useful for monitoring the effect of beta-interferon treatment, and changes in IL-23 and IL-26 should not be ignored as well [17].

In some studies, after four weeks of fingolimod treatment, the percentage of Th17 cells in some patients decreased. In other patients, an increased percentage of Th17 cells was found, which was associated with an onset of the disease [18].

Sato et al. performed a study involving twenty-one patients, monitoring the level of Th17 cells and the ratio of the Th17/Th1 cells during fingolimod treatment for four weeks. They reported that after four weeks in 48% of patients, Th17 cells decreased. The remaining 52% of patients had elevated Th17 cells. The authors reported an increase in Th17/Th1 cells only in one of these patients who had flares. The authors declare that an increase in Th17 cell levels and a Th17/Th1 cell ratio could be associated with the risk of relapse or worsening of the disease symptoms during fingolimod treatment [18].

IL-22 helps to disrupt the blood-brain barrier and facilitate the passage of autoreactive T cells into the CNS. Rolla et al. conducted a study involving 72 patients with relapsing MS who had not received beta-interferon, glatiramer acetate, or immunosuppressant for at least three months. The authors found that levels of Th17 cells increased during the active phase of the disease, whereas an increase in Th22 cells was detected up to a month before the exacerbation, suggesting that the expansion of the latter could be used as a marker for a future worsening of the disease [8].

Th22 cells are involved in various inflammatory processes in the body, including conditions such as psoriasis. Unlike Th17 cells, Th22 lymphocytes are insensitive to beta-interferon. This observation could be one of the reasons for resistance to beta-interferon treatment for the patient population with a higher percent of Th22 lymphocytes.

Moreover, it was shown that Th22 cells and Th17 cells express almost uniformly the IFNAR2 receptors on their surface, whereas Th22 cells have low expression of IFNAR1 receptor. Reduced IFNAR1 levels correlate with a decrease in interferon-β1-related STAT1 phosphorylation and transcription of interferon-β1-related genes. This indicates that unlike Th17 cells, Th22 cells cannot be suppressed by beta-interferon treatment. The authors report that increased production of Th22 cells may be one of the significant factors that increase resistance to beta-interferon therapy [8].

CONCLUSION

Knowing these immunological mechanisms in the pathogenesis of the disease allows examination of specific cells and cytokines to improve the patients' quality of life by control of their therapy, and the possibility of prediction of the risk of relapses.

REFERENCES

[1] Farrell RA. *Neutralizing Antibodies to Interferon Beta in Multiple Sclerosis*. Thesis for doctoral degree, submitted in Department of Neuroinflammation, Institute of Neurology, University College London. 2010; p. 26-69.

[2] Hernandez AL, O'Connor KC, David A, Hafler DA. Multiple sclerosis. In: Mackay IR, Rose NR, editors. *The Autoimmune Diseases*. Academic Press; 2014. p. 735-749.

[3] Georgiev D. Multiple sclerosis and other demyelinating diseases. In: Milanov I, editor. *Neurology*. Sofia: Medicine and Physical Culture; 2012. p. 595-613.

[4] Milanov I. editor. Multiple sclerosis and autoimmune demyelinating diseases of the central nervous system. Sofia: Medicine and Physical Culture; 2014. p. 37-227.

[5] Ireland SJ, Monson NL, Davis LS. Seeking balance: Potentiation and inhibition of multiple sclerosis autoimmune responses by IL-6 and IL-10. *Cytokine*, 2015;73(2):236-44.

[6] Sominanda, A. Interferon-beta-treatment in multiple sclerosis: analysis of neutralizing antibodies. Thesis for doctoral degree, submitted in Division of Neurology Huddinge, Department of Clinical Neuroscience, *Karolinska Institutet*. 2008. 5-9, p. 35-36.

[7] Waldman A, Ghezzi A, Bar-Or A, Mikaeloff Y, Tardieu M, Banwell B. Multiple sclerosis in children: an update on clinical diagnosis,

therapeutic strategies, and research. *The Lancet Neurology.* 2014; 13(9):936-948.

[8] Rolla S, Bardina V, De Mercanti S, Quaglino P, De Palma R, Gned D, Brusa D, Durelli L, Novelli F, Clerico M. Th22 cells are expanded in multiple sclerosis and are resistant to IFN-β. *J. Leukoc. Biol.* 2014;96(6):1155-64.

[9] Myhr KM. Vitamin D treatment in multiple sclerosis. *J. Neurol. Sci.* 2009;286(1-2):104-8.

[10] Passos GR, Sato DK, Becker J, Fujihara K. Th17 Cells Pathways in Multiple Sclerosis and Neuromyelitis Optica Spectrum Disorders: Pathophysiological and Therapeutic Implications. *Mediators Inflamm.* 2016:5314541.

[11] Luchtman DW, Ellwardt E, Larochelle C, Zipp F. IL-17 and related cytokines involved in the pathology and immunotherapy of multiple sclerosis: Current and future developments. *Cytokine Growth Factor Rev.* 2014;25(4):403-13.

[12] Mao P. Reddy PH. Is multiple sclerosis a mitochondrial disease? *Biochim. Biophys. Acta.* 2010;1802(1):66-79.

[13] Shah A, Flores A, Nourbakhsh B, Stüve O. Multiple sclerosis. In: Cifu DX editor. *Braddom's Physical Medicine and Rehabilitation.* Elsevier; 2015. p. 1029-1052.

[14] Waldman A, Ghezzi A, Bar-Or A, Mikaeloff Y, Tardieu M, Banwell B. Multiple sclerosis in children: an update on clinical diagnosis, therapeutic strategies, and research. *The Lancet Neurology.* 2014;13(9):936-948.

[15] Arellano G, Acuña E, Reyes LI, et al. Th1 and Th17 Cells and Associated Cytokines Discriminate among Clinically Isolated Syndrome and Multiple Sclerosis Phenotypes. *Front. Immunol.* 2017; 8:753.

[16] van Langelaar J, van der Vuurst de Vries RM, Janssen M, et al. T helper 17.1 cells associate with multiple sclerosis disease activity: perspectives for early intervention. *Brain.* 2018;141(5):1334-1349.

[17] Esendagli G, Kurne AT, Sayat G, Kilic AK, Guc D, Karabudak R. Evaluation of Th17-related cytokines and receptors in multiple

sclerosis patients under interferon β-1 therapy. *J. Neuroimmunol.* 2013;255(1-2):81-4.

[18] Sato DK, Nakashima I, Bar-Or A, Misu T, Suzuki C, Nishiyama S, Kuroda H, Fujihara K, Aoki M. Changes, and Th17 and regulatory T cells after fingolimod initiation to treat multiple sclerosis. *J. Neuroimmunol.* 2014;268(1-2):95-8.

In: Th17 Cells in Health and Disease
Editor: Tsvetelina Velikova

ISBN: 978-1-53617-152-5
© 2020 Nova Science Publishers, Inc.

Chapter 9

INFLAMMATORY BOWEL DISEASE IN CHILDREN AND ADOLESCENTS: TH17 CELLS AND OTHER PLAYERS

Rayna R. Shentova-Eneva[*], MD, PhD

Department of Gastroenterology and Hepatology,
University Children's Hospital "Prof. Dr. Ivan Mitev," Sofia, Bulgaria
Medical University – Sofia, Bulgaria

ABSTRACT

Inflammatory bowel disease is a heterogeneous group of disorders affecting the intestinal mucosa. Pediatric inflammatory bowel disease is a different disease entity from adult-onset. It differs in many aspects, including the disease type, location of the lesions, disease behavior, and genetically attributable risks. Pediatric-onset inflammatory bowel disease has aggressive disease phenotype, resistance to conventional immunosuppressant therapy, and unique complications. Th17 cells play a role in the pathogenesis of pediatric IBD as well. The condition is always challenging and requires hard teamwork and multidisciplinary approach.

---

[*] Corresponding Author's Email: rshentova@yahoo.com.

152 *Rayna R. Shentova-Eneva*

Keywords: pediatric inflammatory bowel disease, ulcerative colitis, Crohn's disease, Th17 cells, IL-17

INFLAMMATORY BOWEL DISEASES

IBDs is a collective term that includes a group of idiopathic conditions characterized by chronic inflammation of the gastrointestinal tract. The main representatives of this group are Crohn's disease (CD) and ulcerative colitis (UC).

UC is the IBD, which was first described. In 1859, Sir Samuel Wilks (1824-1911) introduced the concept of "ulcerative colitis" to describe the intestinal findings in a deceased young girl [1, 2]. The second half of the nineteenth century contributed to the accumulation of numerous reports of chronic non-infectious diarrhea. In January 1909, at a symposium organized by the Royal Society of Medicine in London, over 300 cases of UC treated at London hospitals were presented and discussed. In the same year, John Percy Lockhart-Mummery (1875-1957) demonstrated that sigmoidoscopy was a safe and invaluable method for colonic evaluation and diagnosis of UC [1]. Over the next decades, knowledge of this disease gradually expanded. Lewisohn demonstrated familial predisposition, Hewitt demonstrated an association between UC and polyps, and Wangensteen demonstrated that this disease is precancerous [1]. In 1923, Helmholtz reported the first cases of UC in children, and in 1949, Warren and Sommers published the first detailed description of the pathomorphological findings in UC, with many photographs and micrographs [1].

The first series of CD cases was published by the Scottish surgeon Thomas Kennedy Dalziel (1861-1924) as early as in 1913 [1]. However, the year of recognition of this disease is considered to be 1932, when a landmark article by Dr. Burrill Crohn (1884-1984) and his colleagues Leon Ginzburg (1898-1988) and Gordon D. Oppenheimer (1900-1974) was published in the October issue of the Journal of the American Medical Association [1, 3]. In this article, they described a condition called

Inflammatory Bowel Disease in Children and Adolescents 153

"regional ileitis" in 14 patients aged from 17 to 52, which later became popular as CD. During the period between 1932 and 1950, this disease was found to occur throughout the gastrointestinal tract. Cases of CD affecting the esophagus, stomach, duodenum, or jejunum were reported. The disease was also found to occur in patients as old as 80 years and older, and young children under ten years of age.

The technological advances in medicine over the years, in particular, the development of fiber optic colonoscopy, which allows taking biopsies, and the ileocolonoscopy, have revolutionized the diagnosis of IBDs worldwide. New bowel imaging methods, such as video-capsule endoscopy, computed tomography enterography, and magnetic resonance enterography, genetic and immunological tests, further extend the diagnostic capabilities and knowledge of IBDs.

Pediatric IBD (PIBD) is defined as having an age of occurrence younger than 17 years. The latest modification of the IBD classification has further classified PIBD into early-onset (EO) IBD when it occurs between 10 and 17 years of age and very-early-onset (VEO) IBD in children younger than 10 years (some consider 6 years), with that diagnosed before 1 year of age called infantile IBD [4, 5].

Currently, the group of IBDs in childhood includes three nosological entities: Crohn's disease, ulcerative colitis and IBD-unclassified [5].

Crohn's Disease

CD is a disease whose predilection site for development is the terminal ileum, but it may affect any part of the gastrointestinal tract, from the mouth to the anus [6]. What is typical of pediatric patients is the more frequent involvement of the colon and the upper gastrointestinal tract compared to adults [7, 8, 9]. According to data from the European Registry of Pediatric Patients with IBD, EUROKIDS, isolated colon involvement is observed in 41% of patients under 10 years of age, and in 27% of older children (colonic form); in 53% of cases the terminal ileum and colon are affected (ileocolonic form), and changes in the esophagus, stomach or duodenum are observed in 30%. Isolated involvement of the terminal ileum occurs in only 16% of cases [10].

The initial macroscopic changes in CD are hyperemia and edema of the affected mucosa, together with the formation of discrete superficial ulcerations – "aphthous lesions." With the progression of the disease, deep ulcers passing transversely and longitudinally across the inflamed mucosa are formed, which gives the musoca the typical cobblestone appearance. The changes are often segmental, the diseased sections alternating with healthy ones - the so-called skip lesions. Inflammation in CD is transmural and may affect the entire bowel wall. Initially, infiltrates are localized around the intestinal crypts, but with the disease progression, deeper layers are involved, and specific histological structures are formed - non-caseating epithelioid granulomas [5, 6, 10, 11]. Granulomas pathognomonic for CD are found in 25% - 75% of cases, with a higher incidence in childhood [12, 13]. Transmural inflammation also predetermines disease-specific complications - wall thickening and narrowing of the lumen of the intestine, intestinal obstruction, fistulation, and abscess formation [10].

Ulcerative Colitis

In UC, inflammatory changes are usually localized in the colonic mucosa. The inflammation is ulcerative and purulent, and it is continuous, generally starting from the rectum and gradually extending to the more proximal parts of the bowel. Histological findings include chronic inflammation of the mucosa with infiltration of polymorphonuclear neutrophils, accumulation of polymorphonuclear neutrophils in the crypts of the large intestine, formation of crypt abscesses, and disruption of the structure of the mucous glands. In more severe cases, inflammatory pseudopolyps are formed. The wall of the intestine becomes thick and rigid, without haustration [5, 6, 11, 14].

Atypical phenotypic manifestation of the disease is common in pediatric patients. There are 5 phenotypes: 1) In 5% to 30% of pediatric patients with UC, no macroscopic involvement of the rectum is found - rectal sparing UC; 2) In patients with short-term disease, usually patients < 10 years of age, it is possible that a continuous course of inflammation may not be observed and typical changes in the architectonics of crypts may be absent; 3) Isolated involvement of the cecum is observed in 2% of the pediatric patients with UC - cecal path; 4) In 4% to 8% of the children with UC, involvement of the upper gastrointestinal tract (GIT) is observed, and in 0.8% of the patients changes are found in the esophagus or duodenum - usually erosions, rarely ulcerations; 5) In the initial clinical manifestation of acute severe ulcerative colitis, it is possible to observe some of the characteristic features of CD, such as deep ulcers and transmural inflammation, which are associated with the severity of the disease. The peculiarities of the phenotypic manifestation of UC in childhood required a revision of the definition of the disease and introduction of two new concepts - typical UC, usually occurring with the involvement of the rectum and subsequently the proximal parts of the colon, and atypical UC, with atypical course without involvement of the rectum, with alternating course of inflammation, with isolated involvement of the cecum, with changes in the upper GIT and/or with deep ulcers and transmural inflammation [14, 15, 16].

IBD-Unclassified

IBD-unclassified is a diagnosis that is made in patients with IBD in whom the inflammation is confined to the colon, and the disease has characteristics that do not allow to determine definitively whether it is UC or CD despite all necessary tests [5, 11, 16, 17, 18].

Indeterminate colitis is a term introduced by pathologists, which is used in cases of colectomy in which definitive diagnosis of UC or CD cannot be made, despite all tests. The inflammatory process is uncharacteristic - there is an overlap of histological signs characteristic of UC with that characteristic of CD [18].

EPIDEMIOLOGY OF PEDIATRIC IBD

Approximately 25% of cases of IBD occur in childhood [19, 20, 21]. In other cases, the clinical manifestation is in adulthood, with a peak in the second and third decades of life [22]. The majority of newly diagnosed pediatric patients are teenagers, but the disease may manifest earlier [7, 23]. Heyman et al. summarised the data from a large multicenter registry comprising 1,739 children with IBD and found that 36.9% of participants were 13-17 years old at diagnosis; 47.7% were 6-12 years old; 15.4% were under 6 years of age, and only 6.1% were under 3 years of age [7]. Lindberg et al. found that of 639 children diagnosed with IBD in Sweden in the period 1984 to 1995, 30.2% were under ten years of age, and according to Kugathasan et al. 20% of all pediatric cases of IBD occur and are diagnosed below ten years of age [17, 24].

The incidence of IBD is variable. Studies carried out in different European countries report an incidence of 0.6-6.8 cases per 100,000 children/year for CD and 0.8-3.6 cases per 100,000 children/year for UC, with a trend of increasing incidence in recent years [25-29]. Generally, UC is more common than CD in pre-school age, whereas, in older children, the incidence of CD is three times higher than the incidence of UC [7, 25, 26, 29]. There is also a slight predominance of male sex in pre-pubertal patients with CD [30, 31]. The incidence of IBD-unclassified is in the range from 5% to 30% [16, 23, 26].

IBDs are considered to be diseases of the so-called "developed countries," and according to some studies, their incidence depends on the gross domestic product of each country [32, 33]. A decreasing north-south gradient of incidence is observed. Data from a prospective study in Europe, including 20 centers, shows that the incidence rate in the Northern countries is 40% higher than in the Countries of the south [34]. The European race is mostly affected. African Americans and Asians are thought to be at lower risk of developing IBD [6]. In the Jewish population, the incidence rate is 2 to 9 times higher than the incidence rate in the general population [35].

ETIOLOGY AND PATHOGENESIS OF PEDIATRIC IBD

The etiopathogenesis of IBDs is not well understood. A number of genetic and immunological factors, as well as specific environmental factors, play a role in their development and manifestation. In childhood, genetic and immune disorders are considered to be of major importance, while environmental factors are predominant in later clinical manifestation [31, 36].

Approximately 25% - 30% of pediatric patients with IBD have at least one relative with such a disease, with familial predisposition being more pronounced in CD. In most cases, the same disease develops [7, 37]. With a first-degree lineal ancestor with CD, the relative risk of developing the disease in the generation is 13-36 times higher than in the general population, and with a first-degree lineal ancestor with UC, the relative risk of developing the disease in the generation is 7-17 times higher than in the general population [38].

There are more than 160 genes associated with the development of IBD, and most of these genes encode different components of the innate or acquired immunity. The *NOD2/CARD15* mutation is one of the earliest identified predispositions for the development of CD. Being a carrier of one risk allele increases the probability of developing the disease by two to four times while being a carrier of two risk alleles increases it by 20 to 40 times. Mutations in the *ATG16L1* and *IRGM* genes related to the autophagy process are also associated with the development of CD. Impairment of the so-called intestinal epithelial barrier genes (*ECM1*, *CDH1*, *NHF4A*, *LAMB1*, and *GNA12*), as well as mutations in the gene encoding the proapoptotic p53 protein, predispose to the development of UC. Other genes associated with the development of IBD are *IBD5*, *IL23-R*, *TL1A*, *IL7R*, *IL8RA/IL8RB*, *DAP*, *LSP1*, and *IRF5* [39, 40].

Some types of infantile IBD or very early onset IBD (VEO IBD) are thought to be a monogenic disease, often involving genes associated with primary immunodeficiency owing to inherited variants that may contribute to dysregulated immunologic homeostasis in the intestine. Identified genetic variants associated with VEO IBD include *ADAM17*, *IKBKG*,

158   *Rayna R. Shentova-Eneva*

COL7A1, *FERMT1*, *TTC7A*, and *GUCY2* [4]. VEO IBD can also be caused by mutations in *IL10*, *IL10RA*, *IL10RB*, *NCF2*, *NCF4*, *XIAP* or *LRBA* [4]. Several other primary immunodeficiency disorders predispose to IBD, including leaky severe combined immune deficiency, bare lymphocyte syndrome, Wiskott-Aldrich syndrome, hyper IgM syndrome, ataxia-telangiectasia, hyper-IgE syndrome, chronic granulomatosis disease, common variable immunodeficiency, and immune dysregulation disorders such as immune dysregulation, poly-endocrinopathy, and enteropathy X-linked (IPEX) syndrome [4].

In older children and adults, genetic factors alone are not sufficient for developing IBD. Of the environmental factors, the following play a more significant role: breastfeeding - as a protective factor; intestinal microflora - dysbiosis is a key predisposing factor to the development of IBD; certain nutritional, viral and bacterial antigens which are considered to be associated with the development of IBD; smoking - a risk factor for development of CD and protective for development of UC; appendectomy - a protective effect for development of UC, and others. [41, 42].

TH17 CELLS IN THE PATHOGENESIS OF PIBD

The multifactorial etiology of IBDs defines their complex pathogenesis. Generally, genetically predisposed individuals are considered to have a defect in their intestinal immune system, which results in the development of a pathological immune response to the contents of the intestinal lumen and environmental factors (intestinal microflora, infectious agents, nutrient antigens, etc.). This defect results in damaging the body's own structures. For example, the product of the *NOD2/CARD15* gene is a protein that plays a role in the intracellular recognition and processing of bacteria and their products. Mutations in *NOD2/CARD15*, as well as changes in *ATG16L1* and *IRGM* genes, lead to "defective" intracellular recognition and processing of bacteria and bacterial products and play a key role in the immunogenetics of Crohn's disease. Mutations in the genes of the intestinal epithelial barrier (*ECM1*,

CDH1, *NHF4A*, *LAMB1*, and *GNA12*) lead to an increase in its permeability, continuous suprathreshold antigenic irritation of the local immune system, and development of a chronic inflammatory process causing UC [39, 40].

Dysbalance in the *IL-23* and *IL-6* signaling pathways also plays an important role in the pathogenesis of PIBD. Both *IL-23* and *IL-6* are pleiotropic cytokines involved in the regulation of the immune response, inflammation, and hematopoiesis. They participate in the development and perpetuation of PIBD by regulating the balance of Treg and Th cells [43]. Serum *IL-23* and *IL-6* levels are increased in the children with IBD and are in positive relationships with other proinflammatory cytokines such as *IL-17A* produced by Th17 cells [43]. The levels of *IL-17* and *IL-23* are elevated in the serum and intestinal mucosa of patients with IBD, and these levels positively correlate with the disease severity [43].

Contrary to the earlier confidence that in immune activation pathways in IBD TH1/TH2 play a dual role, Th17-Treg dysfunction has recently been implicated. Th17 cells are associated with the inflammatory phenotype whereas the regulatory Treg cells are linked to an anti-inflammatory suppressive role [44]. Both Th 17 and Treg cells express a CC motif chemokine receptor 6 (CCR6), a member of the G protein-coupled receptor superfamily, which, upon binding with its chemokine ligand 20 (CCL20), starts the signaling pathway known as classical via the activation of G proteins [44]. The CCR6 expression on Th17 is encouraged by numerous pro-inflammatory cytokines such as *IL-17A-F*, *IL-21*, *IL-22*, *IL-23*, *IL-1β*, *INF-γ*, *IL-6* and tumor necrosis factor-alpha (*TNF-α*) along with the transcription factors retinoic-acid-receptor-related orphan nuclear receptor gamma t (*RORγt*), signal transducer and activator of transcription 3 (*STAT3*) and nuclear factor kappa B (*NF-κB*). CCR6 expression on regulatory Treg cells is induced by transforming growth factor-beta (*TGF-β*) and *IL-10* together with the nuclear receptor forkhead box P3 (*FoxP3*). Experimental studies suggest that Th17 and Treg cells can oscillate between both inflammatory and suppressive roles [44]. In addition, current study in pediatric patients with IBD suggests that Crohn's disease and ulcerative colitis have different pathogenesis mechanisms associated with Th17 cells [45].

Recent data have highlighted the role of *IL-15* and *IL-37* as key players in the pathogenesis of mucosal lesions in pediatric patients with IBD, to a similar extent to *TNF-α* and *INF-γ*. They demonstrated elevated expression of *IL-15* on the epithelial layer of the intestinal mucosa and an increased *IL-37* expression in submucosal lymphoid cells that correlate with histological severity score in young patients with IBD [46].

Various pro- and anti-inflammatory cytokines produced by innate immune cells and T cells are involved in the pathogenesis of PIBD [45]. The cytokine expression pattern is different, depending on the localization of the lesions along the intestine and the specific pathology of the children affected by IBD [47]. Some cytokines are common and target molecules of the new IBD therapies [39, 40, 48,].

CLINICAL PRESENTATION OF PEDIATRIC IBD

The classic symptoms of PIBD are abdominal pain, chronic diarrhea, weight loss, astheno-adynamia, fever, and rectorrhagia. As in adult patients with IBD, the manifestation of the disease is largely related to its location, and the degree of inflammation [49]. The leading symptom for which pediatric patients with UC seek medical attention is bloody diarrhea (90%), and in patients with CD - abdominal pain (70%) [6]. It is important to keep in mind that the classic triad - abdominal pain, diarrhea, and weight loss occurs in only 25% of children with CD [50]. In most cases, quite mild and atypical symptoms are observed, such as malaise, fatigue, and gastric discomfort. However, in some case the opposite is observed - abdominal pain is so severe that it mimics acute appendicitis and children undergo unnecessary surgery [6]. Some symptoms, such as growth retardation and pubertal developmental delay, are typical of childhood and do not occur in adult patients [6]. Growth retardation was observed in 85% of children with CD at the time of diagnosis and in 65% of patients with UC. In 35%

Inflammatory Bowel Disease in Children and Adolescents 161

of cases with CD and 10% of cases with UC, it had preceded the diagnosis by years [49, 51, 52].

Extraintestinal manifestations occur in up to 35% of the cases of IBD in childhood. The following is affected: **bones** - osteopenia, osteoporosis, fractures; **joints** - arthralgia, arthritis, ankylosing spondylitis; **skin** - erythema nodosum, pyoderma gangrenosum, perianal disease, metastatic CD; **eyes** - uveitis, episcleritis, conjunctivitis; **liver** - primary sclerosing cholangitis, hepatitis, cholelithiasis; pancreas - acute pancreatitis; **kidneys** - nephrolithiasis, hydronephrosis, amyloidosis, enterovesical fistula, urinary tract infection; **blood vessels** - vasculitis, propensity for thrombosis; **blood** - iron deficiency anemia, anemia in chronic disease, thrombocytosis, autoimmune hemolytic anemia, vitamin B12 deficiency and others. [6, 49].

DIAGNOSIS OF PEDIATRIC IBD

Diagnosis of IBD in childhood is often a challenge for the treating physician. To unify, assist and facilitate the process, in 2005 in the city of Porto, Portugal, the IBD Working Group of the European Society for Pediatric Gastroenterology, Hepatology and Nutrition [ESPGHAN] introduced and published consensus-based criteria for diagnosing IBD in pediatric patients, the so-called Porto criteria [11].

According to the Porto criteria, the correct diagnosis of PIBD is complex and based on the combination of:

- Medical history: abdominal pain, diarrhea, rectorrhagia, and weight loss, which persist for ≥ four weeks or recurrent symptoms (≥ 2 episodes within six months).
- Physical condition: pale skin, retardation in growth, delay in pubertal development, aphthous changes in the oral mucosa, perianal disease, palpation of an "abdominal mass" or extraintestinal manifestations.

162 *Rayna R. Shentova-Eneva*

- Altered laboratory parameters, such as low hemoglobin and albumin level, thrombocytosis, elevated inflammation markers (ESR, CRP), low iron level, etc. are observed. However, in 21% of children with mild CD and 54% of children with mild UC, the laboratory parameters may be normal [53, 54].
- Serological markers: antibodies against Saccharomyces cerevisiae (ASCA). They are associated with CD and are found in approximately 60% of patients with CD, in 10% of patients with UC and in < 5% of patients with unclassified colitis; the presence of perinuclear anti-neutrophil cytoplasmic antibodies (pANCA). They are associated with UC and are found in approximately 60% of patients with UC, in 20% of patients with CD, and in < 5% of patients with IBD-unclassified [18].
- Ruling out infectious agents and tuberculosis.
- Abdominal ultrasonography - a thickened wall of intestinal loops, changes in vascularization.
- Esophagogastroduodenoscopy (EGD) and ileocolonoscopy (ICS) with multiple biopsies and histology - essential for determining the type of disease, its location, extent, and severity.
- Imaging of small intestine.

The Porto criteria were revised in 2014. The new criteria consist of 12 recommendations, incorporating the Paris modification of the Monreal classification (see below), the original Porto criteria, and consideration of fecal and serum biomarkers [5]. In addition, the group advocated for upper endoscopy for all patients with suspected IBD and the use of small bowel imaging unless the diagnosis favors typical UC. The revised Porto criteria provided an algorithm for assigning the type of IBD, which considers atypical variants of UC and IBDU [5].

Validated, multi-item, scoring systems are used for evaluation of disease activity and severity in pediatric patients with IBD. Pediatric Crohn's Disease Activity Index (PCDAI) is used for measuring disease activity in children and adolescents with Crohn's disease, and Pediatric

Ulcerative Colitis Activity Index (PUCAI) is used for measuring disease activity in children and adolescents with Ulcerative Colitis [55, 56].

CLASSIFICATION OF PEDIATRIC IBD

The need for classification of IBDs arises from the significant differences observed in their clinical presentation and course. Accurate determination of the phenotype of IBD is important for a better understanding of the pathophysiology of its various manifestations, for determining the prognosis and for selecting the most appropriate therapy. For this reason, the Vienna Classification of CD was established in 1998 [57]. Subsequently, the classification was revised and expanded to include UC as well, and in 2005 the Montreal Classification of IBDs was developed [18]. As the Montreal Classification is not able to capture all the characteristics of IBDs in childhood, a group of international experts made its pediatric modification, and in 2009 the Paris Classification was established, which is still used today (**Table 1** and **Table 2**).

The Montreal Classification introduced the diagnosis "unclassified colitis" but did not include it in the classification itself. Subsequently, it was not included in the Paris Classification [58].

A recent study examined the role of histology in determining the phenotype of CD in pediatric patients. The results show that in 56.6% of cases there was a discrepancy between the macroscopic and the microscopic findings, i. e. when histological results are considered, more patients will have ileocolonic location of the disease (L3) rather than isolated involvement of the colon (L2) or terminal ileum (L1) [59]. Despite the eloquent results, it is currently considered that more multicenter studies should be carried out to confirm the need for adding histologic findings to the parameters of the Paris Classification of CD [59].

Table 1. Paris Classification for Crohn's disease [58]

Age at diagnosis	A1a: 0 - <10 y
	A1b: 10 - <17 y
	A2: 17 – 40 y
	A3: > 40 y
Location	L1: distal 1/3 ileum ± limited cecal disease
	L2: colonic
	L3: ileocolonic
	L4a: upper disease proximal to Ligament of Treitz
	L4b: upper disease distal to Ligament of Treitz and proximal to distal 1/3 ileum
Behavior	B1: nonstricturing nonpenetrating
	B2: stricturing
	B3: penetrating
	B2B3: both penetrating and stricturing disease, either at the same or different times
	p: perianal disease modifier
Growth	G0: No evidence of growth delay
	G1: Growth delay

Table 2. Paris Classification for Ulcerative colitis [58]

Extent	E1: ulcerative proctitis
	E2: Left-sided UC (distal to splenic flexure)
	E3: Extensive (hepatic flexure distally)
	E4: Pancolitis (proximal to hepatic flexure)
Severity	S0: never severe[*]
	S1: ever severe[*]

[*] Severe defined by Pediatric Ulcerative Colitis Activity Index (PUCAI) $\geq$65 [56]

CONCLUSION

Pediatric-onset IBD represents a distinct disease with differences in pathogenesis, clinical presentation, disease location, and progression compared with its adult counterpart. The aggressive disease phenotype, resistance to conventional immunosuppressant therapy, and unique complications of PIBD are always challenging and require hard teamwork and a multidisciplinary approach.

REFERENCES

[1] Mulder, D; Noble, A; Justinic, Ch; et al. A tale of two diseases: The history of inflammatory bowel disease. *J Crohns Colitis*, 2014, 8(5), 341-8.

[2] Wilks, S. Morbid appearances in the intestine of Miss Bankes. *Lond Med Gaz*, 1859, 2, 264–265.

[3] Crohn, BB; Ginzburg, L; Oppenheimer, GD. Regional ileitis. A pathologic and clinical entity. *JAMA*, 1932, 99, 1323-9.

[4] Almana, Y; Mohammed, R. Current concepts in pediatric inflammatory bowel disease; IL10/IL10R colitis as a model disease. *Int J Pediatr Adolesc Med.*, 2019, 6(1), 1-5.

[5] Levine, A; Koletzko, S; Turner, D; et al. ESPGHAN revised Porto criteria for the diagnosis of inflammatory bowel disease in children and adolescents. *J Pediatr Gastroenterol Nutr.*, 2014 Jun, 58(6), 795-806.

[6] Mamula, P; Markowitz, JE; Baldassano, RN. *Pediatric Inflammatory Bowel Disease*, Second Edition 2013.

[7] Heyman, MB; Kirschner, BS; Gold, BD; et al. Children with early onset inflammatory bowel disease (IBD): analysis of a pediatric IBD consortium registry. *J Pediatr.*, 2005, 146(1), 35–40.

[8] Shaoul, R; Karban, A; Reif, S; et al. Disease behavior in children with Crohn's disease: the effect of disease duration, ethnicity, genotype; and phenotype. *Dig Dis Sci.*, 2009, 54, 142–50.

[9] Sonnenberg, A; Melton, SD; Genta, RM. Frequent occurrence of gastritis and duodenitis in patients with in fl ammatory bowel disease. *In fl amm Bowel Dis.*, 2011, 17, 39–44.

[10] De Bie, CI; Buderus, S; Sandhu, BK; et al. Diagnostic workup of paediatric patients with inflammatory bowel disease in Europe:

results of a 5-year audit of the EUROKIDS registry. *J Pediatr Gastroenterol Nutr.*, 2012, 54(3), 374-80.

[11] IBD Working Group of the European Society for Paediatric Gastroenterology, Hepatology and Nutrition. Inflammatory bowel disease in children and adolescents: recommendations for diagnosis-- the Porto criteria. *J Pediatr Gastroenterol Nutr.*, 2005, Jul, 41(1), 1- 7.

[12] Potzi, R; Walgram, M; Lochs, H; et al. Diagnostic significance of endoscopic biopsy in Crohn's disease. *Endoscopy.*, 1989, 21, 60-62.

[13] Satsangi, J; Sutherland, LR; Colombel, JF. Inflammatory bowel disease. *Churchill Livingstone*, 2003.

[14] Levine, A; de Bie, CI; Turner, D; et al. EUROKIDS Porto IBD Working Group of ESPGHAN. Atypical Disease Phenotypes in Pediatric Ulcerative Colitis: 5-year Analyses of the EUROKIDS Registry. *Inflamm Bowel Dis*, 2013, 19, 370–377.

[15] Rajwal, SR; Puntis, JW; McClean, P; et al. Endoscopic rectal sparing in children with untreated ulcerative colitis. *JPGN*, 2004, 38, 66–69.

[16] Carvalho, RS; Abadom, V; Dilworth, HP; et al. Indeterminate colitis: a significant subgroup of pediatric IBD. *Inflamm Bowel Dis.*, 2006, 12(4), 258–262.

[17] Lindberg, E; Lindquist, B; Holmquist, L; Hildebrand, H. Inflammatory bowel disease in children and adolescents in Sweden, 1984-1995. *J Pediatr Gastroenterol Nutr.*, 2000, 30(3), 259-64.

[18] Satsangi, J; Silverberg, MS; Vermeire, S; Colombel, JF. The Montreal classification of inflammatory bowel disease: controversies, consensus, and implications. – *Gut and liver.*, 2006, 55(6), 749-753.

[19] Auvin, S; Molinie, F; Gower-Rousseau, C; et al. Incidence, clinical presentation and location at diagnosis of pediatric infl ammatory bowel disease, a prospective population-based study in northern France (1988-1999). *J Pediatr Gastroenterol Nutr.*, 2005, 41, 49-55.

[20] Baldassano, RN; Piccoli, DA. In fl ammatory bowel disease in pediatric and adolescent patients. *Gastroenterol Clin North Am.*, 1999, 28, 445–58.

[21] Braegger, CP; Ballabeni, P; Rogler, D; et al. Epidemiology of Infl ammatory Bowel Disease: Is There a Shift Towards Onset at a Younger Age? *J Pediatr Gastroenterol Nutr.*, 2011, 53, 141-144.

[22] Binder, V. Epidemiology of IBD during the twentieth century: an integrated view. *Best Pract Res Clin Gastroenterol.*, 2004, 18, 463-479.

[23] Mamula, P; Telega, GW; Markowitz, JE; et al. Inflammatory bowel disease in children 5 years of age and younger. *Am J Gastroenterol.*, 2002, 97, 2005-2010.

[24] Kugathasan, S; Judd, RH; Hoffmann, RG; et al. Epidemiologic and clinical characteristics of children with newly diagnosed inflammatory bowel disease in Wisconsin: a statewide populationbased study. *J Pediatr.*, 2003, 143(4), 525–31.

[25] Henderson, P; Hansen, R; Cameron, FL; et al. Rising incidence of pediatric infl ammatory bowel disease in Scotland. *Infl amm Bowel Dis.*, 2012 Jun, 18(6), 999-1005.

[26] Hildebrand, H; Finkel, Y; Grahnquist, L; et al. Changing pattern of paediatric infl ammatory bowel disease in northern Stockholm 1990-2001. *Gut.*, 2003, 52, 1432-1434.

[27] Jakobsen, C; Paerregaard, A; Munkholm, P; et al. Pediatric infl ammatory bowel disease: increasing incidence, decreasing surgery rate, and compromised nutritional status: A prospective population-based cohort study 2007-2009. *Infl amm Bowel Dis.*, 2011, 17, 2541-2550.

[28] Karolewska-Bochenek, K; Lazowska-Przeorek, I; Albrecht, P; et al. Epidemiology of infl amatory bowel disease among children in Poland. A prospective, population-based, 2-year study, 2002-2004. *Digestion.*, 2009, 79, 121-129.

[29] Sawczenko, A; Sandhu, BK; Logan, RF; et al. Prospective survey of childhood inflammatory bowel disease in the British Isles. *Lancet.*, 2001, 357, 1093-1094.

[30] Biank, V; Broeckel, U; Kugathasan, S. Pediatric inflammatory bowel disease: clinical and molecular genetics. *Inflamm Bowel Dis.*, 2007, 13, 1430-1438.

[31] Bousvaros, A; Sylvester, F; Kugathasan, S; et al. Challenges in pediatric inflammatory bowel disease. *Inflamm Bowel Dis.*, 2006, 12, 885-913.

[32] Mayberry, JF. Some aspects of the epidemiology of ulcerative colitis. *Gut*, 1985, 26(9), 968–974.

[33] Mayberry, JF; Rhodes, J. Epidemiological aspects of Crohn's disease: a review of the literature. *Gut*, 1984, 25(8), 886–899.

[34] Shivananda, S; Lennard-Jones, J; Logan, R; et al. "Incidence of inflammatory bowel disease across Europe: is there a difference between north and south? Results of the European collaborative study on inflammatory bowel disease (EC-IBD). *Gut*, 1996, 39 (5), 690–697.

[35] Duerr, RH. The genetics of inflammatory bowel disease. *Gastroenterol Clin North Am.*, 2002, 31, 63–76.

[36] Cuffari, C. Diagnostic Considerations in Pediatric Inflammatory Bowel Disease Management. *Gastroenterol Hepatol* (N Y)., 2009 Nov, 5(11), 775–783.

[37] Weinstein, TA; Levine, M; Pettei, MJ; et al. Age and family history at presentation of pediatric inflammatory bowel disease. *J Pediatr Gastroenterol Nutr.*, 2003, 37, 609-613.

[38] Laharie, D; Debeugny, S; Peeters, M; et al. Inflammatory bowel disease in spouses and their offspring. *Gastroenterology.*, 2001, 120, 816–9.

[39] Lees, CW; Barrett, JC; Parkes, M; Satsangi, J. New IBD genetics: common pathways with other diseases. *Gut.*, 2011 Dec, 60(12), 1739-53.

[40] Shih, DQ; Targan, SR; McGovern, D. Recent advances in IBD pathogenesis: genetics and immunobiology. *Curr Gastroenterol Rep.*, 2008 Dec, 10(6), 568-75.

[41] Kugathasan, S; Amre, D. Infl ammatory bowel disease-- environmental modification and genetic determinants. *Pediatr Clin North Am.*, 2006, 53, 727-749.

[42] Molodecky, N; Kaplan, G. Environmental Risk Factors for Inflammatory Bowel Disease. *Gastroenterol Hepatol* (N Y)., 2010 May, 6(5), 339–346.

[43] Zhu, XM; Shi, YZ; Cheng, M; Wang, DF; Fan, JF. Serum IL-6, IL-23 profile and Treg/Th17 peripheral cell populations in pediatric patients with inflammatory bowel disease. *Pharmazie.*, 2017 May 1, 72(5), 283-287.

[44] Ranasinghe, R; Eri, R. CCR6–CCL20 Axis in IBD: What Have We Learnt in the Last 20 Years? *Gastrointest. Disord.*, 2018, 1, 57-74.

[45] Cho, J; Kim, S; Yang, DH; Lee, J; Park, KW; Go, J; Hyun, CL; Jee, Y; Kang, KS. Mucosal Immunity Related to FOXP3+ Regulatory T Cells, Th17 Cells and Cytokines in Pediatric Inflammatory Bowel Disease. *J Korean Med Sci.*, 2018, Dec 10, 33(52), e336.

[46] Vitale, S; Strisciuglio, C; Pisapia, L; Miele, E; Barba, P; Vitale, A; Cenni, S; Bassi, V; Maglio, M; Del Pozzo, G; Troncone, R; Staiano, A; Gianfrani, C. Cytokine production profile in intestinal mucosa of paediatric inflammatory bowel disease. *PLoS One.*, 2017, Aug 10, 12(8), e0182313.

[47] Verdier, J; Begue, B; Cerf-Bensussan, N; Ruemmele, FM. Compartmentalized expression of Th1 and Th17 cytokines in paediatric inflammatory bowel diseases. *Inflamm Bowel Dis.*, 2012, 18(7), 1260–6.

[48] Annaházi, A; Molnár, T. Pathogenesis of Ulcerative Colitis and Crohn's Disease: Similarities, Differences and a Lot of Things We Do Not Know Yet. *J Clin Cell Immunol*, 2014, 5, 253.

[49] Mamula, P; Markowitz, JE; Baldassano, RN. Inflammatory bowel disease in early childhood and adolescence: special considerations. *Gastroenterol Clin North Am.*, 2003, 32, 967-995.

[50] Sawczenko, A; Sandhu, BK. Presenting features of inflammatory bowel disease in Great Britain and Ireland. *Arch Dis Child.*, 2003, 88, 995-1000.

[51] Kim, SC; Ferry, GD. Inflammatory bowel diseases in pediatric and adolescent patients: clinical, therapeutic, and psychosocial considerations. *Gastroenterology.*, 2004, 126, 1550-1560.

[52] Seidman, E; Leleiko, N; Ament, M; et al. Nutritional issues in pediatric inflammatory bowel disease. *J Pediatr Gastroenterol Nutr.*, 1991, 12, 424-438.

[53] Cabrera-Abreu, JC; Davies, P; Matek, Z; et al. Performance of blood tests in diagnosis of inflammatory bowel disease in a specialist clinic. *Arch Dis Child.*, 2004, 89, 69-71.

[54] Mack, DR; Langton, C; Markowitz, J; et al. Laboratory values for children with newly diagnosed inflammatory bowel disease. *Pediatrics.*, 2007, 119, 1113-1119.

[55] Hyams, JS; Ferry, GD; Mandel, FS; Gryboski, JD; Kibort, PM; Kirschner, BS; Griffiths, AM; Katz, AJ; Granel, RJ; Boyle, JT; Michener, WM; Levy, JS; Lesser, ML. Development and validation of a pediatric Crohn's disease activity index. *J Pediatr Gastroenterol Nutr*, 1991, (12), 439 – 447.

[56] Turner, D; Otley, AR; Mack, D; Hyams, J; De Bruijne, J; Uusoue, K; Walters, TD; Zachos, M; Mamula, P; Beaton, DE; Steinhart, AH; Griffiths, AM. Development, validation, and Evaluation of a Pediatric Ulcerative Colitis Activity Index: A Prospective Multicenter Study. *Gastroenterology*, 2007, (133), 423-432

[57] Gasche, C; Scholmerich, J; Brynskov, J; et al. A simple classification of Crohn's disease: report of the Working Party for the World Congresses of Gastroenterology, Vienna 1998. *Inflamm Bowel Dis*, 2000, 6, 8–15.

[58] Levine, A; Griffiths, A; Markowitz, J; et al. Pediatric Modification of the Montreal Classification for Inflammatory Bowel Disease: The Paris Classification. *Inflamm Bowel Dis*, 2011, 17, 1314–1321.

[59] Fernandes, MA; Verstraete, SG; Garnett, EA; Heyman, MB. Addition of Histology to the Paris Classification of Pediatric Crohn Disease Alters Classification of Disease Location. *J Pediatr Gastroenterol Nutr.*, 2016 Feb, 62(2), 242-5.

In: Th17 Cells in Health and Disease
Editor: Tsvetelina Velikova

ISBN: 978-1-53617-152-5
© 2020 Nova Science Publishers, Inc.

Chapter 10

TH17/TREGS CELLS IN PATIENTS WITH ULCERATIVE COLITIS DURING ANTI-TNFα THERAPY

Tsvetelina Velikova[1], MD, PhD,
Ekaterina Ivanova-Todorova[1,*], MD, PhD,
Zoya Spasova[2], MD, PhD, Maria Petkova[2], MD,
Ekaterina Krasimirova[1], MD, PhD,
Kalina Tumangelova-Yuzeir[1], PhD,
Georgi Vasilev[1], MD, Lyudmila Mateva[2], MD, PhD
and Dobroslav Kyurkchiev[1], MD, PhD

[1]Laboratory of Clinical Immunology, University Hospital
"St. Ivan Rilski," Department of Clinical Immunology,
Medical University of Sofia, Sofia, Bulgaria
[2]Clinic of Gastroenterology, University Hospital "St. Ivan Rilski,"
Department of Internal Medicine, Medical University, Sofia, Bulgaria

---

* Corresponding Author's Email: katty_iv@yahoo.com.

ABSTRACT

Introduction: The dynamic changes between Th17 cells, T effectors (activated Teffs), and Treg subpopulations determine the development of inflammation in chronic inflammatory bowel diseases. Recently, data on the effect of anti-TNFα therapy on Th17/Teffs/Tregs subsets have been accumulated, mainly for Crohn's disease.

Aim: To monitor Th17/Tregs for one year in patients with ulcerative colitis (UC) during anti-TNFα therapy.

Methods: Th17, Teffs, and Tregs in peripheral blood were analyzed by flow cytometry in eight UC patients (before therapy, on the week 6th, on the 3rd month, on the first year) and fifteen healthy controls. All patients on anti-TNFα treatment were followed-up immunologically and clinically.

Results: We found that before therapy, the mean percentage of Th17 lymphocytes in patients was lower than in healthy subjects (8.42% vs. 15.3%, resp.). During the treatment, the patients increased their Th17 level, however, without reaching the mean percentage found in healthy subjects. Regarding Tregs, their percentage was lower before treatment compared to healthy subjects (5.2% vs. 8.9%, resp.). Six patients showed a significant increase in Tregs (mean 11.22%) at the end of the first year, while two patients did not demonstrate such an effect. The described changes correlated with the course of the disease. During the therapy there was a decrease in Teffs in the three patients with established clinical improvement and rise of Teffs in the patient without clinical remission.

Conclusion: Our results demonstrated that biological therapy with anti-TNFα agents affects Th17, Teffs, and Treg subsets, and the changes in these subsets could be predictable for the patients about the response to anti-TNFα therapy.

Keywords: Th17 cells, T effector cells, Tregs, anti-TNFα therapy, ulcerative colitis, IBD

INTRODUCTION

Inflammatory bowel disease (IBD) refers to a group of digestive tract diseases in which the colon and/or small intestine are affected by inflammatory processes. The two main types of conditions that fall into this group are Crohn's disease (CD) and ulcerative colitis (UC) [1]. IBD is a socially significant disease. The active phase is of different duration and may be aggravated by local and systemic complications, some of which are life-threatening [2]. The incidence of IBD is increasing. It is highest in North America and Northern Europe (considered to be diseases of industrialized nations with a high socio-economic standard) - about 7 per 100,000. It is lower in Southern Europe, South Africa, and Australia - about 0.9-3.1 per 100,000. Accurate data on the incidence of both diseases lack in Bulgaria [3]. The peak of the disease is in the second and third decades, but it is also the second smaller peak in patients between the ages of 60 and 70. The white race is more likely to develop the condition [4].

Despite significant progress in recent years, the etiology of inflammatory bowel disease is still unknown. Increasing evidence supports the thesis that IBDs are due to a defect in the intestinal immune system (so-called mucosal immunity). In genetically predisposed individuals, environmental factors, autoimmune, infectious, alimentary, and psychosocial factors are assumed to trigger and maintain a persistent inflammatory response in the intestinal mucosa [5]. The central role of environmental factors is played by the commensal intestinal flora [6], which interacts most closely with structures that are subject to inflammatory changes, and genetic predisposition manifests as a defect in the innate and acquired immunity, mucosal barrier function and permeability and cellularity mucosal. The NOD2/CARD15 (or IBD1) gene localized on chromosome 16, predisposing to Crohn's disease, has been identified [7].

The picture described in IBD is related to the acute inflammation, which usually resides within hours to days as the neutrophils themselves live [8]. Neutrophils, on the one hand, can assist tissue repair [10] and, on the other, assist in the maintenance of inflammation and mucosal remodeling by their ability to secrete TNFα. Locally active cytokines TNFα and IL-1β can enter the bloodstream and exert their systemic effects - hyperpyrexia, appetite suppression, inducing cachexia [8], C-reactive protein (CRP) secretion, general fatigue.

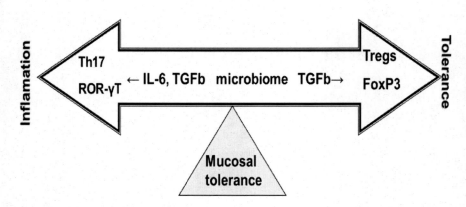

Figure 1. The relation between inflammation, tolerance, and microbial flora for developing oral mucosal tolerance.

The reciprocal interaction between T regulatory (Tregs) and Th17 lymphocytes makes it possible to alter the balance between them to restore and promote tolerance in IBD [9], as well as in other autoimmune diseases. Moreover, the dynamics between Th17, Teffs (activated T effectors), and Treg cells determine the development of inflammatory process in chronic IBD. Recently, data on the effect of anti-TNFα therapy on Th17/Teffs/Tregs subsets have been accumulated, mainly for patients with Crohn's disease.

Th17 cells and Treg cells are found on surfaces, where they exert barrier functions and protect the organism via two mechanisms - from pathogens or excessive T-cell immune reactions. Despite the seemingly opposite service, both cells share a common pattern of development, which is regulated by TNFα, IL-6, retinoic acid, and the microbiome.

In short, IBD is characterized by a breakdown in the intestinal homeostasis and chronic intestinal inflammation through various cytokine pathways (Figure 1).

An alternative to severe and treatment-resistant IBD is the so-called biological therapy. It is based on the use of drugs directed against specific molecules or mediators that play a crucial role in the inflammation process (such as TNFα). Monoclonal antibodies against TNFα have been developed and researched widely. Before initiation, like the treatment with immunosuppressants, it is necessary to exclude the presence of systemic infections such as tuberculosis, chronic hepatitis, etc. However, it is recommended to follow-up on the therapy with biological drugs. The development of therapeutic strategies with monoclonal antibodies against specific cytokines or subunits and receptors that are important for differentiation, maintenance or secretion of Th17 cells are promising in patients with this type of immune-mediated disease, as well as for finding clinically useful markers for the diagnosis and follow-up of patients with IBD.

AIM OF THE STUDY

To detect the changes in Th17 cells, T effectors, and T regulatory cells, we aimed to monitor the percentages of Th17/Teffs/Tregs in peripheral blood of patients with UC during anti-TNFα therapy for one-year-period.

DESIGN OF THE STUDY

We performed a one-year immunological monitoring of UC patients on anti-TNFα therapy. The study included patients with two types of anti-TNFα mAb: Golimumab and Adalimumab.

Blood samples from eight UC patients and fifteen healthy volunteers were used for detection of Th17, T effector, and Treg cells in peripheral blood:

- Prior to initiation of treatment with anti-TNFα;
- At the 6th week of onset of therapy;
- At the 3rd month;
- On the 1st year of treatment.

Table 1. Baseline characteristics of the UC patients

Variable	N (%), or Median (range)
Disease localization	
Pancolitis	5 (62%)
Proctosigmoiditis	3 (38%)
Duration of the disease, years	11,71 ± 7,23 (4-22)
Mayo score	>10
Medications at baseline	
5-ASA	1
Corticosteroids + 5-ASA	1
Azathioprine + 5-ASA	4
Azathioprine/MTX + 5-ASA + Corticosteroids	2
Medication during anti-TNFα therapy	
5-ASA	1
Corticosteroids + 5-ASA	1
Azathioprine + 5-ASA	4
Azathioprine/MTX + 5-ASA + Corticosteroids	2
Anti-TNFα - subcutaneous administration	
Golimumab	4 (50%)
Adalimumab	4 (50%)

PARTICIPANTS AND METHODS

Participants

Eight adult UC patients (four males and four females) at mean age 48.25 years (36-68) were prospectively included. All of them were considered to have a clinical indication for anti-TNFα therapy, according to the recommended inductive protocol. The patients were previously diagnosed for UC based on clinical, biological, endoscopic, and histological signs of the disease according to the ECCO guidelines (2017). The other baseline characteristics of the patients are presented in Table 1.

Fifteen healthy controls at mean age 34.06 years (28-43) were also recruited for comparison, analyzing their peripheral blood.

Clinical response to anti-TNFα treatment was defined as a decrease in the Mayo score below 2. Clinical response or remission was evaluated at 6th week, 3rd month, and one year after the first anti-TNFα infusion. All patients were monitored for drug levels and antibodies against anti-TNFα mAb. All patients had proper therapeutic levels of the drug and did not develop antibodies against anti-TNFα.

The protocol was approved by local EC (Ethical Committee), and all participants signed written inform consent before including in the study.

Methods

We performed flow cytometric determination of the percentage of lymphocyte subpopulations in peripheral blood. Th17 cells were defined by expressing the markers CD3+CD4+CD161+CD196(CCR6)+ simultaneously and expressed as a percentage of CD4+ T lymphocytes.

Tregs were assessed by the expression of the transcription factor FoxP3 from T helper cells groups and defined as CD3+CD4+CD25hi+/-FoxP3+.

Teffs were examined from the CD4+T lymphocytes as expressing the following markers CD3+CD4+CD25+FoxP3-.

RESULTS

We found that these patients who were responders exerted significantly increased percentages of Tregs among total CD4+ T cells was after one year on anti-TNFα therapy compared to those percentages before treatment (Figure 2).

This upregulation in Tregs percentage was due mainly at the raise of the CD4+FoxP3+CD25- T cells. The two clinical non-responders were Tregs non-responders, too, and we observed a decrease in % of Tregs population (Figure 2). The mean percentage of Treg cells in peripheral blood of UC patients remain lower than those of the healthy controls before anti-TNFα, while at the first year of therapy in responders, Tregs were significantly higher than before the treatment (Figure 3).

We also found that before therapy, the mean percentage of Th17 lymphocytes in the peripheral blood of UC patients was lower than by healthy subjects (8.42% vs. 15.3%). During treatment, the patients raised the level of their Th17 cells, but they remained below the mean percentage found in healthy subjects (Figure 4). Only one patient showed a sharp increase in the percentage of the Th17 cells, but by the end of the first year, Th17 cells were normalized to the level of healthy controls.

At the end of the first year of treatment, the levels of Th17 were reduced in those patients who also had clinical remission with Mayo score less than two. In only two patients (i.e., the non-responders), Th17 cells were increased sharply during treatment. In one patient, it was observed acute severe recurrence disease with endoscopic data of pancolitis, and in the other - active proctitis was found.

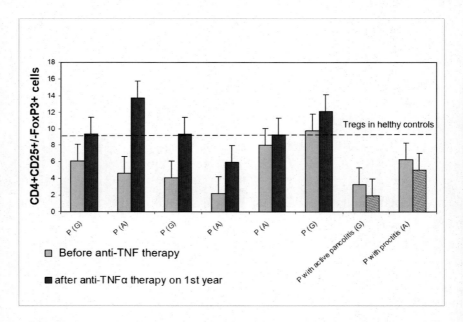

Figure 2. The percentage of Tregs before and after anti-TNFα treatment.

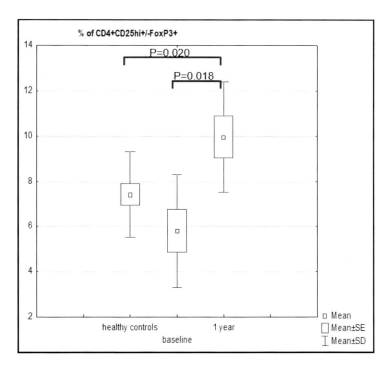

Figure 3. At the first year of anti-TNFα therapy, Tregs were considerably higher than before the treatment in responders.

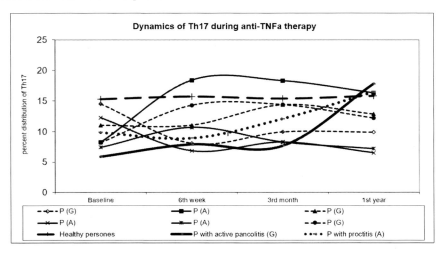

Figure 4. The dynamics of Th17 cells in UC patients before and after anti-TNFα therapy.

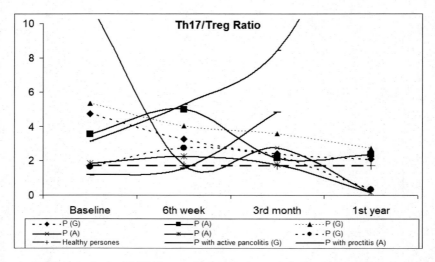

Figure 5. Changes in the Th17/Treg ratio during the anti-TNFα in responders and non-responders of UC patients.

Our results also demonstrated that before treatment, the Th17/Treg ratio was higher than this observed the healthy controls and gradually declined in the first year of therapy related to anti-TNFα therapy in responders. In non-responders, the Th17/Treg ratio was evaluated as progressively increased directly related to the severity of the disease (Mayo score<2) (Figure 5).

We found that in patients who responded to therapy that there is a significant downregulation in CD4+CD25+FoxP3- Teffs on the first year related to the severity of the disease as well (Figures 6 and 7).

DISCUSSION

Anti-TNFα therapy may lead to a significant rise in the number of peripheral blood Tregs in patients responding to this therapy. They may induce the differentiation of a population of iTregs from CD4+CD25-FoxP3+ cells. We choose to determine the CD25hi+ and CD25- but all FoxP3+ T helper cells because there is unequivocal evidence that the FoxP3 transcription factor is a major player for the suppressor functions of

Tregs. In addition, there is new evidence that CD3+CD4+CD25-FoxP3+ cells are precursors to CD3+CD4+CD25hi+FoxP3+ Tregs [10].

The observed lower Tregs percentages for patients with pre-treated UC compared to healthy controls are probably due to duration of the disease above ten years and immunosuppression (AZA/MTX). This suggests that over time, the number of FoxP3+ T cells may decrease.

Meanwhile, Th17 cells in patients with UC before anti-TNFα administration were lower than average in the healthy subjects. Probably the reason is the extended immunosuppressive therapy. During the treatment, the patients show increased Th17 levels but below the mean percentage found in healthy subjects. One possible explanation is that treatment with TNFα inhibitors can result in several outcomes, including the induction of specific T cell subsets such as Tregs or Th17 cells [11].

Our findings are following the investigation of Bischetti et al. [12] who found lower Tregs in active IBD (both Crohn`s disease and UC) in comparison with the healthy controls (2.8% ± 0.4% vs. 4.6% ± 0.6%, respectively; p = 0.01).

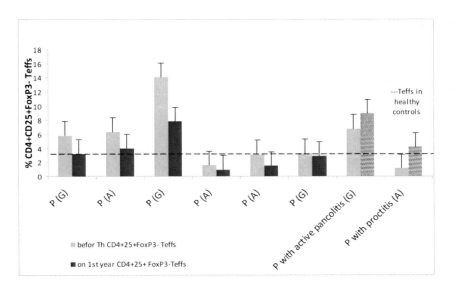

Figure 6. Downregulation of CD4+CD25+FoxP3- Teffs on the first year of anti-TNFα therapy related to the severity of the disease in patients with UC.

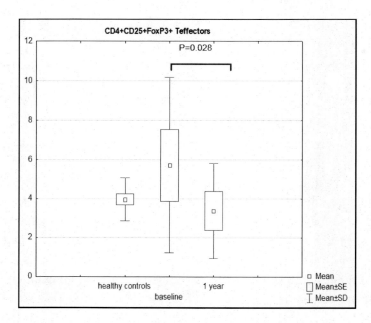

Figure 7. CD4+CD25+FoxP3+ Teffs in the first year of anti-TNFα therapy in patients with UC.

Furthermore, Tregs were similarly decreased in the blood of CD patients (3.1% ± 0.4%) and UC patients (2.5% ± 0.6%; p = 0.3) [12].

However, a single exposure to anti-TNFα therapy was associated with a significant increase in the percentage of CD4+CD25+Foxp3+ cells in 4/5 of patients with IBD patients by the end of the second week (from 4.0% ± 0.5% to 2.8% ± 0.4%; p = 0.001) compared to the pretreatment percentages [12]. They also reported that three out of five patients, peripheral Treg cells did not change after anti-TNFα treatment, although they had an excellent clinical response to treatment after six weeks [12].

Our results also demonstrated that the Th17/Tregs ratio in UC patients before anti-TNFα therapy is higher than in healthy subjects, which is directly related to the severity of the disease (Mayo score <2). At the end of the first year after anti-TNFα therapy, the patients which Th17/Tregs ratio reduced and Tregs were increased, we observed clinical and endoscopic remission.

The obtained results are not surprising; they agree with previous studies showing that active IBD exerts a selective defect in circulating CD4+CD25+Foxp3+T cells. This defect could be only partly compensated for by a rise in Foxp3+T cells in the lamina propria of the inflamed mucosa in the gut.

Several mechanisms may have contributed to the potentiation of Tregs by anti-TNFa therapy. Firstly, treatment with monoclonal antibodies against TNFα could have encouraged the survival of Tregs, for example, by reducing the rate of apoptosis. Secondly, the quantitative increase of Tregs expressing upregulated levels of Foxp3+ and the related suppressive function could be a result of activation and proliferation of preexisting Foxp3+ Tregs or because of their differentiation by conversion from Foxp3 precursors [13, 14].

Thirdly, although anti-TNFα agents inhibit Treg function at a high dose, exposure to a low dose of anti-TNFα treatment instead promotes activation, survival, and expansion of Tregs. This is achieved by signaling via high-affinity receptor TNFRII of Tregs. It may be guessed that whereas anti-TNFα monoclonal antibodies may neutralize serum TNFα efficiently, the access into the inflamed mucosa is more limited. Therefore, antibodies might allow binding of residual TNFα to Tregs and to enhance their survival and functions. There is a lot of evidence to assume that Tregs contribute to the efficacy of anti-TNFα monoclonal antibodies therapy. Furthermore, the renewal of Treg cells follows the anti-TNFα therapy-induced recovery of intestinal homeostasis [15, 16].

We can also speculate that the increase of Tregs and the decrease of CD4+CD25+FoxP3- Teffs at the same time may serve as a predictive factor of response to anti-TNFα therapy.

We have to take into account the prevalence of circulating IL-17 and Foxp3+ CD4+ T cells, which are increased in patients with IBD. Coexpression of RORγt and Foxp3 in these cells denotes the possible conversion from both Treg cells to Th17 cells and vise verse. This is associated with a decreased suppressive function of Foxp3 CD4+ T lymphocytes in patients with IBD [17]. We did not assess this problem, and this is one of our study limitations.

CONCLUSION

This chapter contributes to the accumulation of more and better knowledge in the field of immunopathogenesis and therapy for patients with UC based on changes in the axis of Th17 cells and Tregs relationship.

Our findings demonstrated that anti-TNFα therapy might lead to a significant rise in the number of peripheral blood Tregs and decrease in activated Teffs in patients that respond clinically to treatment. In line with this, the increase of Tregs and the decrease to CD4+CD25+FoxP3- Teffs simultaneously may be useful as a predictive factor of response to biological therapy.

REFERENCES

[1] Longo D, Fauci A, Kasper D, Hauser S, Jameson J, Loscalzo J. *Harrison's Principles of Internal Medicine*. 17th ed.

[2] Velikova T, Miladinova R, Ivanova-Todorova E, et al. Extraintestinal Manifestations and Intestinal Complications in Patients with Crohn's Disease: Associations with Some Clinico-Laboratory Findings, Immunological Markers, and Therapy, *Acta Medica Bulgarica*, 2018,45(1), 16-21.

[3] Diagnostic and therapeutic algorithm (consensus) of the Bulgarian Scientific Society of Gastroenterology. Chronic inflammatory bowel disease, ulcerative colitis and Crohn's disease. Bulgarian *Hepatogastroenterology*, Book 2, 2010, 47-55.

[4] Satsangi J, Silverberg MS, Vermeire S, Colombel JF. The Montreal classification of inflammatory bowel disease: controversies, consensus, and implications. *Gut and liver*. 2006;55(6):749-753.

[5] Hisamatsu T, Kanai T, Mikami Y, Yoneno K, Matsuoka K, Hibi T. Immune aspects of the pathogenesis of inflammatory bowel disease. *Pharmacology & Therapeutics*. 2013;137(3):283-297.

[6] Chung H, Kasper DL. Microbiota-stimulated immune mechanisms to maintain gut homeostasis. *Current Opinion in Immunology.* 2010;22(4):455-460.

[7] Robertson SJ, Zhou JY, Geddes K, et al. Nod1 and Nod2 signaling does not alter the composition of intestinal bacterial communities at homeostasis. *Gut Microbes.* 2013;4(3):222-231.

[8] McDonald T. Immunology and Diseases of the Gut 2006.

[9] Velikova T, Kyurkchiev D, Spassova Z, et al. Alterations in cytokine gene expression profile in colon mucosa of Inflammatory Bowel Disease patients on different therapeutic regimens. *Cytokine.* 2017;92:12-19.

[10] Vukmanovic-Stejic M, Zhang Y, Cook JE et al. Human CD4+ CD25hi Foxp3+ regulatory T cells are derived by rapid turnover of memory populations *in vivo. J. Clin. Invest.* 2006;116(9): 2423-2433.

[11] Bystrom J, Clanchy FI, Taher TE et al., TNFa in the regulation of Treg and Th17 cells in rheumatoid arthritis and other autoimmune inflammatory diseases. *Cytokine* 2016;101:4-13.

[12] Boschetti G, Nancey S, Sardi F. Therapy with anti-TNFα antibody enhances number and function of Foxp3(+) regulatory T cells in inflammatory bowel diseases. *Inflamm. Bowel Dis.* 2011;17(1):160-70.

[13] Heetun Z, Doherty GA. Restoring the Regulatory Regime in IBD: Do Anti-TNF Agents Rescue Treg? *Inflammatory Bowel Diseases* 2012, 18(6):1186-1187.

[14] Veltkamp C, Anstaett M, Wahl K, et al. Apoptosis of regulatory T lymphocytes is increased in chronic inflammatory bowel disease and reversed by anti-TNFα treatment. *Gut* 2011;60(10):1345-53.

[15] Guidi L, Felice C, Procoli A, et al. FOXP3+ T Regulatory Cell Modifications in Inflammatory Bowel Disease Patients Treated with Anti-TNF Agents. *BioMed. Research International* 2013;2013, Article ID 286368, 10 pages.

[16] Liu C, Xia X, Wu W et al. Anti-tumour necrosis factor therapy enhances mucosal healing through down-regulation of interleukin-21

expression and T helper type 17 cell infiltration in Crohn's disease. *Clin. Exp. Immunol.* 2013;173(1):102-11.

[17] Ueno A, Jijon H, Chan R et al. Increased prevalence of circulating novel IL-17 secreting Foxp3 expressing CD4+ T cells and defective suppressive function of circulating Foxp3+ regulatory cells support plasticity between Th17 and regulatory T cells in inflammatory bowel disease patients. *Inflamm. Bowel Dis.* 2013;19(12):2522-34.

In: Th17 Cells in Health and Disease
Editor: Tsvetelina Velikova

ISBN: 978-1-53617-152-5
© 2020 Nova Science Publishers, Inc.

Chapter 11

TH17 CELLS INVOLVEMENT IN CELIAC DISEASE

Gergana Taneva[1], and Tsvetelina Velikova[2]*
[1]Sveta Sofia Hospital, Sofia, Bulgaria
[2]Clinical Immunology, University Hospital Lozenetz,
Sofia University, Sofia, Bulgaria

ABSTRACT

Gluten enteropathy (GE, a.k.a. celiac disease) is an autoimmune disease that affects the small intestine in a genetically predisposed individual, caused by immunological hypersensitivity to gluten. Th1 and Th17 cells seem to play a central role in the pathogenesis of the disease. The current understanding suggests that HLA-DQ protein complex induces Th1 response, and increased production of cytokines, especially IFNγ, leads to intestinal mucosa damage. However, evidence suggested the ambiguous role of Th17 in immune responses observed in GE, where the exact function of IL-17A in GE pathogenesis is still debated and open to investigation, the cytokine may be involved in refractory GE. Anti-cytokine therapy and gluten-vaccines could be proposed as promising effective treatment options for patients with GE in the future.

---

[*] Corresponding Author's Email: gergana.taneva@mail.bg.

Keywords: gluten enteropathy, celiac disease, Th17 cells, IL-17, anti-tTG, anti-DGP, gluten, vaccine

INTRODUCTION

Gluten enteropathy (GE, a.k.a. celiac disease) is an autoimmune disease that affects the small intestine in a genetically predisposed individual and is caused by immunological hypersensitivity from the toxic action of gluten [1]. The incidence of GE has increased significantly over the last 50 years, with the majority of patients remaining undiagnosed. The diagnosis is based on clinical, serological and histological studies. The treatment of the disease is a gluten-free diet. Patients need to be well-informed about the risks of complications and the need for follow-up [2]. The main trigger factor of the disease is an environmental factor - gluten exposure. Loss of gluten tolerance can occur at any age and can be triggered by other factors, such as gastrointestinal infections, medications, surgery and more [3].

Gluten-related disorders become an epidemiological problem. The spectrum of these disorders includes neurological, skin, etc. autoimmune diseases, as well as an increased risk of malignancies. Gluten and gluten-related proteins are wide-spread in food industry – they can be found in barley, wheat, rye, oats, and many processed foods. Gluten is a mixture of vegetable proteins (prolamines and gluten) [4, 5].

Over the last 50 years, diagnosis and screening of patients at risk were improved. However, most of the affecting people fall under the peak of the statistical iceberg, and many of them remain undiagnosed [2].

In western countries, the incidence of GE is approximately 0.6% (histologically confirmed) and 1% (serologically proven). It affects all age groups, with 70% of patients being diagnosed under 20 years of age. The incidence of the disease is higher in patients with other autoimmune disorders or patients with first and second-line relatives suffering from GE [6].

GENETIC FACTORS IN CELIAC DISEASE

The most common known human leukocyte antigens (HLA) haplotypes in people with GE are HLA DQ 2.5, HLA DQ8 (rarely), and HLA DQ2.2 (the rarest). Having this genetic factor means that the patient may develop celiac disease in their life. In 95% of patients with celiac disease, the haplotypes DR3-DQ2 are detected and in the remaining 5% - DR4-DQ8. Homozygous female carriers have a higher risk of celiac disease development than males or heterozygous carriers [7]. Genetic testing may be helpful in cases where celiac disease is diagnosed, but the gluten-free diet does not improve the symptoms [7]. It could also be useful to estimate personal risk assessment.

The absence of HLA-DQ2/8 rejects the diagnosis of celiac disease and in the presence of gastrointestinal symptoms and manifestations of malabsorption (chronic diarrhea, steatorrhea, weight loss, swelling, flatulence, postprandial abdominal pain) directs to the search for another enteropathy.

Susceptibility to developing GE can be inherited, but not the disease itself. The reason for that is because GE is a multifactorial disorder, where multiple genes interact with environmental factors to cause GE. However, there are also non-HLA genes that are less understood [8]. Therefore, GE can run in families, but there is no specific inheritance pattern.

The risk mentioned above for a relative of an affected person to develop GE is mostly based on empiric risk data that has been reported. The child's overall risk for GE is 5-10% if the genetic status is not known. After genetic testing of the susceptibility genes, the risk will increase or decrease depending on the results [9].

PATHOGENESIS OF GLUTEN ENTEROPATHY

After entering the lumen of the small intestine, gliadin is digested by border enzymes to amino acids and peptides. Tissue transglutaminase (tTG) is a calcium-dependent enzyme that catalyzes the hydrolysis, or so-called deamidation (conversion of the amino acid glutamine to glutamate). Gliadin is rich in glutamine and is a specific substrate for tTG [2].

tTG selectively deamidates gliadin molecules that enter the lamina propria of the mucosa. The gliadin complex associated with tTG forms a neoantigen, which is presented by HLA-DQ2 and recognized by intestinal T-helper (CD4+) cells. This process is not observed in healthy individuals. Gluten - sensitive CD4+ T cells activate and Th1 immune response occurs, associated with T - bet transcription factor activation and production of large amounts of IFNg leading to inflammation and mucosal damage [2].

The peptides, formatted after the selective deamidation of gliadin by the action of intestinal tTG in the mucosa, are called deamidated gliadin peptides (DGPs) [2]. DGPs can bind with high affinity to HLA DQ2 or DQ8 on antigen-presenting cells of GE patients followed by stimulation of further inflammatory responses in the small intestines [1]. This process of selective deamidation of gliadin results in a dramatic increase in the sensitivity and specificity of the anti-DGP antibodies [10]. Other celiac-related antibodies are anti-F-actin antibodies (AAA). They show the degree of villous atrophy, where the main component of cytoskeleton microfilaments – actin, is affected [11]. It was also demonstrated that the measurement of anti-DGP antibodies in serum is an excellent predictive marker with high diagnostic accuracy for GE [12].

TH17 CELLS AND CELIAC DISEASE

Patients with GE have expanded CD4+ T cell clones that are specific to gluten peptides, to tTG, to DGP and actin. After recognition of gluten by Th1 lymphocytes, a robust immune response develops, leading to intestinal damage and manifested symptoms of the disease. Patients who start gluten-free diet report for reduction in clinical symptoms, whereas the histological features such as villous atrophy, intestinal permeability, and crypt hyperplasia are shown to improve [14-17]. The deamidated peptides derived after the activity of the tTG enzyme are detected by T lymphocytes during the deamination process leading to formation of anti-DGP antibodies [18]. The deamidation process increases the ability of the gliadin peptides to bind the HLA-DQ2/8 molecules of antigen-presenting cells and to stimulate Th1, Th2, and Th17 cells. This, in turn, leads to the secretion of pro-inflammatory cytokines (i.e., IFN-γ, IL21, etc.) and the production of more autoantibodies [13, 19].

IL-17A-producing T cells that are involved in the GE pathogenesis secrete IFN-γ [20]. Interestingly, the expression of IL-21 in CD4+ T cells is also increased. Therefore, IL-21 increases IFN-γ production through positive feedback and has important role in the expansion of Th17 cells [21]. It is thought that IL-21 may be involved in promoting intraepithelial CD8+ T cells and celiac-related autoantibody production since IL-21 regulate Bcl-6 expression in B cells [21]. In 2010, Bood and colleagues [22] demonstrated that major source of IL-17 is not gliadin-specific CD4+T cells but other gluten-specific IL-17A-producing cells observed in the duodenum of GE patients [21, 22]. In fact, the authors showed that gluten- reactive T cells produce insignificant amounts of IL-22 [22]. However, another study indicated that both IL-17 and IL-21 have a role in mucosal immunity; therefore, the crucial part for Th17 cells in the pathogenesis of GE has been emphasized again [23, 24]. Furthermore, it was indicated that gliadin-specific Th17 cells also produce the pro-inflammatory cytokines IFN-γ and IL-21, the mucosa-protective IL-22, and TGF-β. This evidence suggests that in GE, Th17 cells secrete both pro-inflammatory and anti-inflammatory cytokines, showing functional plasticity [24].

Several studies also showed that TGF-β is required as a critical signaling cytokine in Th17 differentiation [25]. However, since TGF-β signaling pathways have an essential role in the development of both T regulatory and Th17 cells, low concentration of TGF-β with elevated IL-6 leads to differentiation of Th17 instead of Tregs. Therefore, the differentiation to Th17 or Tregs depends on the cytokines in the microenvironment of intestines. However, in GE, it was demonstrated that

TGF-β activity is impaired due to secretion of IL-15; thus, the differentiation is mainly towards the Th17 cells [25, 26, 27].

DIAGNOSIS AND CLINICAL ASPECTS OF THE DISEASE

GE can be manifested with various complaints - diarrhea, steatorrhea, and weight loss, delayed development of children, abdominal pain, upper-dyspeptic symptoms, and even depression, osteoporosis, infertility, and lymphoma development. The clinical picture is accompanied by laboratory detected deficiencies of iron, vitamin B12, folic acid, anemic syndrome, changes in electrolytes, increased levels of transaminases, decreased absorption of fat-soluble vitamins. In children, the symptoms are more often related to growth retardation, diarrhea, loss of muscle mass, decreased appetite, abdominal discomfort, emotional instability, etc. [28, 29].

The classic form of GE occurs between the 6th and 18th months of the newborn's life and is characterized by chronic diarrhea and malabsorption, anorexia, enlargement of the abdomen, reduction of muscles, accompanied by progressive growth retardation.

The other, or so-called non-classical forms of GE are:

1. Atypical – mostly with extraintestinal complaints.
2. Quiet form - patients have typical morphological changes in the mucosa but have no clinical symptoms.
3. Latent GE - individuals with a genetic predisposition for GE and positive serology, but without changes in the mucosa and without clinical symptoms [30].

GE in adults is usually a non-classical form of the disease.

Aside from the clinical presentation, the presence of autoantibodies, specific for GE, is a crucial part of the diagnosing process. The most common antibodies, their specificity, and sensitivity [12, 28] are shown in Table 1.

Table 1. Celiac-related autoantibodies used in diagnosing process

Antigen	Antibody type	Sensitivity, %	Specificity, %
Gliadin	IgA	85	90
	IgG	80	80
Endomysium	IgA	95	99
	IgG	80	97
Tissue transglutaminase	IgA	98	98
	IgG	70	95
Deamidated gliadin peptide	IgA	88	90
	IgG	80	98

The gold standard for diagnosis is the histological examination and verification and serological confirmation by testing for autoantibodies related to GE. However, 1/3 of patients have no endoscopic changes. If the disease is suspected, it is necessary to take biopsies, even from intact mucosa (at least four), including the duodenal bulb. There are GE cases where the disease may be limited and affect the segment only in bulb duodenum [30]. Highly sensitive and specific endoscopic and histological findings in GE are villous atrophy, nodular mucosa (mosaicism), vascular reduction, etc. [31].

It was shown that the degree of mucosal damage correlates well with serological findings. Evidence indicates that anti-tTG antibodies levels above 100 IU/ml or more correlate with severe villous changes observed in children and adults. Normalizing the mucous membrane may take between six months and one year after starting the gluten-free diet, but the recovery may take more in some patients. After one year, 75% of patients achieve histological remission, but elevated levels of intraepithelial lymphocytes may remain high. Normal levels of anti-TG2 antibodies do not guarantee histological improvement [28].

Since IgA deficiency affects up to 3% of patients with GE, testing for anti-DGP IgG along with anti-tTG IgG antibodies is recommended. In case of IgA deficiency, it is also feasible to search for other causes of intestinal atrophy, such as giardiasis, small intestinal bacterial overgrowth, other immunodeficiency syndromes, etc. [32].

In some patients, positive serology along with negative histology was observed. Although false-positive results for the presence of anti-tTG antibodies are possible, in most cases, these results are due to very low or undetectable titers of antibodies. Causes for false-positive serology are hypergammaglobulinemia, autoimmune diseases, chronic liver diseases, infections. It is essential to verify whether the patients are on a gluten-free diet and if this is the case, they have to be switched off the diet for two to six weeks patients and then retested. In these cases, testing for HLA-DQ2/8 is recommended, if not yet performed [33].

However, up to 15% of patients with GE are seronegative. It can be observed at the onset of the disease but most often when tested again after strict adherence to a gluten-free diet [33]. Since most of the autoantibodies are pathological and lead to mucosal damage, it is essential to desire their levels below the established cut-off.

Our previous findings on celiac-serology showed that the average serum levels of anti-tTG, anti-DGP, anti-gliadin, and AAA were at significantly higher levels in patients with GE compared to healthy persons ($p < 0.001$) [34]. We also observed that the serum level of IL-17A was about 70 times higher in patients with GE than in healthy persons ($p = 0.027$). Our results pointed out anti-DGP antibodies as the most accurate diagnostic test for GE with the highest diagnostic sensitivity of 100%, followed by AGA and anti-tTG antibodies [34]. Although the diagnosis of GE relays on biopsy, our results confirmed that immunological serological testing could be employed with advantages in diagnosis and monitoring of these patients.

When obtain the results from the histological examination, it is recommend to exclude other diseases leading to mucosal atrophy - infectious diseases, nutritional hypersensitivity, peptic ulcer, gastro-duodenitis associated with Helicobacter pylori infection, other autoimmune diseases, HIV, microscopic colitis, bacterial overgrowth syndrome, colitis, use of some medication - PPI, NSAIDs, amyloidosis, eosinophilic gastroenteritis, etc. [35-38].

TREATMENT OF GLUTEN ENTEROPATHY

The well-established and effective treatment for GE is the gluten-free diet. Patients should be instructed not to consume food containing or contaminated with gluten. The menu should be compensated, to be high in fibers. Gluten levels should not exceed 10 – 30 mg since this was shown as the maximum amount that does not cause changes in the duodenal mucosa. Patients, both children and adults who are not on gluten-free diet or do not follow it strictly are prone to increased risk of developing metabolic syndrome, decreased bone density, cardiovascular disease, infertility, causes of miscarriage, etc. [39].

Iron deficiency is observed in seven to 80% of patients with GE; intravenous recovery is required in patients with more severe disease or non-responding to oral therapy with iron medications. It is necessary to take Vitamin B12 and folates, which leads to an improvement in the depressive state and anxiety. Vitamin B12 deficiency is observed in 5–41% of patients. Vitamin D absorption is also impaired due to malabsorption of fat, and also due to the decreased intake of dairy products in these patients [40]. Magnesium and zinc could also be supplemented if needed.

About 40% of patients are overweight and 13% are obese. Most gluten-free foods have a high glycemic index and fats but lower protein levels. Potential risk in these patients is the development of metabolic syndrome and liver steatosis [40].

In a small percentage of patients, the disease can be severe with rapid disease progression and so-called celiac crisis. These patients have acute diarrheal syndrome; they are hemodynamically unstable, with dehydration, neurological manifestations, renal failure, metabolic acidosis, hypoalbuminemia, dyselectrolycemia, significant weight reduction. Hospital treatment with parenteral nutrition and corticosteroid therapy is required [41]. However, this condition is observed very rarely.

In refractory cases of GE, where the gluten-free diet does not improve the clinical course, the use of Budesonide is discussed. The latter helps to alleviate the clinical symptoms in 90% of patients but does not change the histological picture. The combination of Budesonide with Azathioprine, as well as other immunosuppressive drugs - Infliximab, Jak3 inhibitors, brentuximab, and others, is also discussed. At this stage, most experience is gained for the treatment with Budesonide at recommended doses of 3x3mg/day [41].

The risk of malignancies in patients with GE is considerable. Patients who are refractory to the therapy are prone to developing lymphoproliferative diseases and malignancies of the gastrointestinal tracts [42]. The most common intestinal T cell lymphoma related to GE is enteropathy-associated T-cell lymphoma (EATL) type-I [42].

Recently, we published a study on twelve patients on gluten-free-diet whose autoantibodies, along with IL-17 levels, were assessed before and after 12 months on a diet. All patients with initial high IL-17A and anti-tTG levels remained above the upper limit of detection for both parameters. We can hypothesize that high levels of IL-17A could be implemented in the pathogenesis of refractory GE. Our results showed that higher IL-17 and anti-tTG levels are stable in time and could be used as a prognostic factor for patients with refractory GE [43].

ASSOCIATED WITH CELIAC DISEASE SYNDROMES

It is essential to examine not only patients with a typical clinical picture but also those with atypical manifestations of the disease including extraintestinal. These patients could be divided into the following groups:

- Group 1 - patients with atypical symptoms - chronic diarrhea unaffected by treatment, weight loss, developmental delay, vomiting, abdominal pain, amenorrhea, cramps, chronic constipation, aphthous stomatitis, fractures, increased cytolytic enzymes.
- Group 2 - asymptomatic patients at increased risk for GE - Patients with Down syndrome, Turner syndrome, or autoimmune diseases, IgA deficiency, relatives of patients with GE.

Some GE-associated diseases require special attention during the diagnosing process [28]. These diseases of are enlisted below.

Dermatitis Herpetiformis

It is considered a skin manifestation of a disease associated with gluten hypersensitivity. Dermatitis herpetiformis (DH) is characterized by itchy papulovesicular eruptions symmetrically located on the elbows, knees, waist, face, neck, and less often around the mouth. The pathogenesis of DH is associated with pathognomic IgA deposits in the dermis. In the skin of patients with DH, the target for IgA deposition is epidermal transglutaminase -tTG3. Skin lesions are thought to involve neutrophils, which accumulate in the dermis papillae and, by contacting IgA deposits, release their enzymes and inflammatory mediators, which lead to tissue damage and the formation of characteristic lesions. IgA deposits against TG2are detected in the mucosa of the small intestine in patients with GE. The diagnose process includes testing of anti-tTG2 antibodies and histological examination from skin lesions [28]. Although the diagnosis of DH relies on skin histology testing, recently, we showed that the serologic testing of a panel of celiac-related antibodies along with IL-17A levels could be employed with advantages in the diagnosing process of DH patients. We also demonstrated that DH patients with positive serology could have routine monitoring for gut complications typical for GE [44].

Psoriasis

GE is observed in 1-4% of patients with psoriasis. It is thought that vitamin D deficiency, Th1/Th17 abnormal response, genetic factors, and increased intestinal permeability contribute to the disease progression [28].

Neurological Abnormalities

Neurological symptoms that accompanied GE may be associated not only with impaired nutrients absorption. Gluten can cause neurological damage itself through a variety of mechanisms - cross-reacting antibodies, immune complexes and direct toxic effects on the nervous system [28]. Neurological symptoms include dysregulation of autonomic nervous system, cerebellar ataxia, developmental delays, depression, gluten encephalopathy, peripheral neuropathy, etc. Patients with gluten ataxia (that is described as progressive cerebellar injury with generalized muscle weakness and loss of sensitization) have antibodies to gliadin both in the intestine and in the brain.

Once again we want to emphasize the importance of serological testing by citing a clinical case of a 40-year-old Caucasian woman diagnosed with GE in early age, on a gluten-free diet. The diagnosis was serologically and histologically proven after she has been on a common diet for the last decade. Following a new administration on a gluten-free diet, the patient has improved significantly with a marked decrease in the antibodies (anti-tTG and anti-DGP antibodies). Antibodies in the blood can be used for follow-up and measurement of the gluten-free diet compliance, and possibly for prognosis of refractory disease and further complications [45]

SPECIFIC TREATMENT OPTIONS – CELIAC VACCINE AND ANTI-IL-17 DRUGS

Currently, there are no FDA-approved therapeutic options for the treatment of GE except the gluten-free diet. However, recently, a breakthrough was made by constructing a vaccine for GE patients, which mechanism of action is similar to injection of insulin for diabetes. These new approaches promise to treat patients with the disease in the future

Vaccine for Celiac Disease

The Nexvax2 development is part of the epitope-specific immunotherapy for GE. It is a form of immunotherapy, where starting from a small amount of gluten, then gradually increased, aiming patients who possess HLA-DQ2.5 to build up resistance to the gluten. The idea behind the vaccine is the activation of the immune system, especially the part with recognition of gluten as a dangerous substance, to be ceased, then reprogramed to stimulate immune tolerance towards gluten [46]. The desired effect is consuming gluten-containing food, avoiding unfavorable adverse effects. The subtle mechanisms include reprogramming of the T-cells, however, are not fully elucidated [46].

The Phase I trial evaluated the safety, tolerability, and bioactivity of the vaccine. It was also demonstrated an excellent biological response to the included peptides and satisfying safety profile of the vaccine [4]. Phase I trial of Nexvax2-specific T-cell response confirmed the desired bioactivity in HLA-DQ2 genotype patients. The investigations also indicate that the vaccine uses the correct peptides for establishing tolerance towards gluten, especially at the highest doses [47, 48].

Anti-IL-17 Treatment for Celiac Disease Patients

At this point, no clinical trials are known for investigation of Secukinumab as a treatment for GE patients, but in patients with Crohn`s disease and psoriasis. The results were disappointing [49].

CONCLUSION

In general, some critical aspects of the immune pathogenesis of GE have been identified. The adaptive immune system comprises of CD4+ T cell (Th1, Th17 cells) seems to play a central role in the pathogenesis of the disease. The current understanding suggests that HLA-DQ protein complex induces Th1 response, which includes increased production of cytokines, especially IFNγ, leading to intestinal mucosa damage. However, evidence suggested the role of Th17 in immune responses observed in GE, as well as the plasticity actions in GE pathogenesis. The exact function of IL-17A in GE pathogenesis is still debated and open to investigation, the cytokine may be involved in refractory GE. Anti-cytokine therapy and gluten-vaccines could be proposed as promising effective treatment options for patients with GE in the future.

REFERENCES

[1] Kaswala, DH; Veeraraghavan, G; Kelly, CP; et al. *Celiac Disease Diagnostic Standards and Dilemmas Diseases*, 2015, 3, 86-101.

[2] Dias, JA; Port, J. Celiac Disease: What Do We Know in 2017? *GE Gastroenterol*, November 2017, 24, 275-278.

[3] Shannahan, S; Leffler, DA. Diagnosis and Updates in Celiac Disease. *Gastrointest Endosc Clin N Am*, 2017, 27, 79-92.

[4] Green, PHR; Cellier, C; Rubio-Tapia, A; et al. Celiac Disease. *N Engl J Med*, 2007, 357, 1731-43.

[5] Celiac Disease. *Curr Opin Gastroenterol*, 2010, 26, 116-122.

[6] Daniel, A; Leffler, et Schuppan D. Update on Serologic Testing in Celiac Disease. *Am J Gastroenterol*, 2010, 105, 2520–2524.

[7] Taylor, AK; Lebwohl, B; Snyder, CL. Celiac Disease. *Gene Reviews.*, September 17, 2015, http://www.ncbi.nlm.nih.gov/books/ NBK1727/. Accessed 26/10/2019.

[8] Celiac disease. *Genetics Home Reference.*, October, 2011, http://ghr.nlm.nih.gov/condition/celiac-disease.

[9] Alessio, F. Genetics of Celiac Disease. In: Bruce Buehler. *Medscape*, 2012, http://emedicine.medscape.com/article/1790189-overview. Accessed 26/10/2019.

[10] Vermeersch, P; Geboes, K; Mariën, G; et al. Diagnostic performance of IgG anti-deamidated gliadin peptide antibody assays is comparable to IgA anti-tTG in celiac disease. *Clinica Chimica Acta*, 2010, 411, 931-935.

[11] Granito, A; Muratori, P; Cassani, F. Anti-actin IgA antibodies in severe coeliac disease;" *Clin Exp Immunol*, 2004, 137(2), 386-392.

[12] Velikova, TS; Altankova, I. Antibodies against deamidated gliadin peptides in the diagnosis of celiac disease. *Int Med*, 2019, 1(1), 15-18.

[13] Faghih, M; Barartabar, Z; Nasiri, S; et al. The role of Th1 and Th17 in the pathogenesis of celiac disease. *Gastroenterol Hepatol Open Access.*, 2018, 9(2), 83-87.

[14] lid, LM; Steinsbø, Ø; Qiao, S. Small bowel, celiac disease and adaptive immunity. *Dig Dis.*, 2015, 33(2), 115–121.

[15] Escudero-hernández, C; Peña, AS; Bernardo, D. Immunogenetic pathogenesis of celiac disease and non-celiac gluten sensitivity. *Current Gastroenterology Reports.*, 2016, 18(7), 36.

[16] Pagliari, D; Urgesi, R; Frosali, S; et al. The interaction among microbiota, immunity, and genetic and dietary factors is the condicio sine qua non celiac disease can develop. *J Immunol Res.*, 2015, 2015, 123653.

[17] Mazzarella, G. Effector and suppressor T cells in celiac disease. *Word J Gastroenterol.*, 2015, 21(24), 7349–7356.

[18] Wal, Y Van De; Kooy, Y; Veelen, P Van; et al. Cutting edge: selective deamidation by tissue transglutaminase strongly enhances gliadin-specific t cell reactivity. *J Immunol.*, 1998, 161(4), 1585–1588.

[19] Hu, S; Mention, J; Monteiro, RC; et al. A direct role for NKG2D/MICA interaction in villous atrophy during celiac disease. *Immunity.*, 2004, 21(3), 367–377.

[20] Monteleone, I; Sarra, M; Del Vecchio Blanco, G; et al. Characterization of IL-17A-producing cells in celiac disease mucosa. *J Immunol.*, 2010, 184(4), 2211–2218.

[21] Leeuwen, MA Van; Lindenbergh-kortleve, DJ; Raatgeep, HC; et al. Increased production of interleukin-21, but not interleukin-17A, in the small intestine characterizes pediatric celiac disease. *Mucosal Immunol.*, 2013, 6(6), 1202–1213.

[22] Bodd, M; Tollefsen, S; et al. HLA-DQ2-restricted gluten-reactive T cells produce IL-21 but not IL-17 or IL-22. *Mucosal Immunol.*, 2010, 3(6), 594–601.

[23] Blaschitz, C; Raffatellu, M. Th17 cytokines and the gut mucosal barrier. *Journal of Clinical Immunology.*, 2010, 30(2), 196–203.

[24] Eyerich, S; Eyerich, K; Pennino, D; et al. Th22 cells represent a distinct human T cell subset involved in epidermal immunity and remodeling. *Journal of clinical investigation.*, 2009, 119(12), 3573–3585.

[25] Vriezinga, SL; Schweizer, JJ; Koning, F; et al. Coeliac disease and gluten-related disorders in childhood. *Nat Rev Gastroenterol Hepatol.*, 2015, 12(9), 527–536.

[26] Bettelli, E; Carrier, Y; Gao, W; et al. Reciprocal developmental pathways for the generation of pathogenic effector TH17 and regulatory T cells. *Nature.*, 2006, 441(7090), 235–238.

[27] Abadie, V; Sollid, LM; Barreiro, LB; Jabri, B. Integration of genetic and immunological insights into a model of celiac disease pathogenesis. *Annu Rev Immunol.*, 2011, 29(1), 493-525. doi:10.1146/annurev-immunol-040210-092915.

[28] Al-Toma, A; Volta, U; Auricchio, R; et al. European Society for the Study of Coeliac Disease (ESsCD) guideline for coeliac disease and other gluten-related disorders. *United European Gastroenterology Journal*, 2019, 7, 5, 583-613.

[29] Szajewska, H; Shamir, R; Chmielewska, A; et al. Systematic review with meta-analysis: early infant feeding and coeliac disease--update 2015. *Aliment Pharmacol Ther.*, 2015, 41(11), 1038-1054.

[30] Lebwohl, B; Rubio-Tapia, A; Assiri, A; et al. Diagnosis of celiac disease. *Gastrointest Endosc Clin N Am.*, 2012, 22(4), 661-677.

[31] van der Windt, DA; Jellema, P; Mulder, CJ; et al. Diagnostic Testing for Celiac Disease Among Patients With Abdominal Symptoms. *JAMA.*, 2010, 303(17), 1738.

[32] Fasano, A. Clinical presentation of celiac disease in the pediatric population. *Gastroenterology*, 2005, 128(4 SUPPL.1), S68-73.

Th17 Cells Involvement in Celiac Disease 203

[33] Virta, LJ; Kaukinen, K; Collin, P. Incidence and prevalence of diagnosed coeliac disease in Finland: results of effective case finding in adults. *Scand J Gastroenterol.*, 2009, 44(8), 933-938.

[34] Velikova, TS; Spassova, ZA; Tumangelova-Yuzeir, KD; et al. Serological Update on Celiac Disease Diagnostics in Adults. *International Journal of Celiac Disease*, 2018, 6(1), 20-25.

[35] Marsh, MN; Johnson, M; Rostami, K. Mucosal histopathology in celiac disease: a rebuttal of Oberhuber's sub-division of Marsh III. *Gastroenterol Hepatol from bed to bench.*, 2015, 8(2), 99-109.

[36] Corazza, GR; Villanacci, V. Coeliac disease. *J Clin Pathol.*, 2005, 58(6), 573-574.

[37] Adelman, DC; Murray, J; Wu, TT; et al. Measuring Change In Small Intestinal Histology In Patients With Celiac Disease. *Am J Gastroenterol.*, 2018, 113(3), 339-347.

[38] Villanacci, V; Ceppa, P; Tavani, E; et al. Coeliac disease: the histology report. *Dig Liver Dis.*, 2011, 43 Suppl 4, S385-95.

[39] Penagini, F; Dilillo, D; Meneghin, F; et al. Gluten-Free Diet in Children: An Approach to a Nutritionally Adequate and Balanced Diet. *Nutrients.*, 2013, 5(11), 4553-4565.

[40] Hughey, JJ; Ray, BK; Lee, AR; et al. Self-reported dietary adherence, disease-specific symptoms, and quality of life are associated with healthcare provider follow-up in celiac disease. *BMC Gastroenterol.*, 2017, 17(1), 156.

[41] Jamma, S; Rubio-Tapia, A; Kelly, CP; et al. Celiac crisis is a rare but serious complication of celiac disease in adults. *Clin Gastroenterol Hepatol.*, 2010, 8(7), 587-590.

[42] Wierdsma, NJ; Nijeboer, P; Schueren, MA; et al. Refractory celiac disease and EATL patients show severe malnutrition and malabsorption at diagnosis. *Clin Nutr.*, 2016, 35(3), 685-691.

[43] Velikova, TS; Spassova, ZA; Tumangelova-Yuzeir, KD; et al. Higher serum IL-17A along with anti-tTG antibodies for prediction of refractory celiac disease, *GJBAHS*, 2019, 8, 9.

[44] Velikova, TS; Shahid, M; Ivanova-Todorova, E; et al. Celiac-Related Autoantibodies and IL-17A in Bulgarian Patients with Dermatitis

Herpetiformis: A Cross-Sectional Study. *Medicina* (Kaunas)., 2019, 55(5), 136.

[45] Velikova, TS; Taneva, G; Chourchev, S; Tankova, L; et al. A Case Report of a Patient with Gluten Enteropathy: The Importance of Immunological Markers for Diagnosis and Followup" *ARC Journal of Hepatology and Gastroenterology.*, 2018, 3(1), 22-24.

[46] Velikova, Ts. Celiac Disease Vaccination: Expectations and Reality. *J Mucosal Immunol Res*, 2018, 2, e 105.

[47] Celiac News Letter; A Vaccine for Celiac Disease 2017, accessed at https://www.beyondceliac.org/celiac-disease/vaccine/ 26/10/2019.

[48] Celiac Foundation; *A Promising Celiac Disease Drug is moving into Phase II Clinical Trial.* (2017) last accessed at https://celiac.org/about-the-foundation/featured-news/2017/11/promising-celiac-disease-drug-moving-phase-ii-clinical-trial/ on 26/10/2019.

[49] Hueber, W; Sands, BE; Lewitzky, S; et al. Secukinumab in Crohn's Disease Study Group. *Gut*, 2012, 61, 1693–1700.

In: Th17 Cells in Health and Disease
Editor: Tsvetelina Velikova

ISBN: 978-1-53617-152-5
© 2020 Nova Science Publishers, Inc.

Chapter 12

TH17 CELLS AND OTHER PATHOLOGIES

Tsvetelina Velikova, MD, PhD*
Clinical Immunology, University Hospital Lozenetz,
Medical Faculty, Sofia University,
Sofia, Bulgaria

ABSTRACT

The pathogenesis of many inflammatory, allergic, autoimmune, and tumor diseases are assumed to depend on activated T cells, including Th17 cells. The role of IL-17 and Th17 in different pathways has also changed the perspective of immunology regarding the basis of chronic tissue inflammation. The existing concepts of immunopathologic mechanisms related to Th17 cells in allergy, autoimmunity, skin disease, nervous system, and carcinogenesis are extended further in the last decades and have been supported by some studies. Interestingly, Th17 cells exhibit similar behaviors in most diseases where they are considered to play a role. Furthermore, the number of conditions influenced by Th17 cells appears to be increasing. However, in most of them, the exact mechanism of actions of Th17 cells remain unclear, though evidence suggests that they could also play an essential role in the control of these diseases.

---

* Corresponding Author's Email: tsvelikova@medfac.mu-sofia.bg.

Keywords: Th17 cells, IL-17, autoimmunity, allergy, inflammation, blistering skin diseases, multiple sclerosis, cancerogenesis

INTRODUCTION

The pathogenesis of various inflammatory, allergic, autoimmune, and tumor diseases are assumed to depend on activated T cells. The discovery of recently novel T cell subsets that produce IL-17–producing cells, allows us to understand T-cell biology and explain the immunopathogenesis of many disorders [1]. The role of IL-17 and Th17 in different pathways has also changed the perspective of immunology regarding chronic tissue inflammation, particularly when other T-helper cells cannot explain. The existing concepts of immunopathologic mechanisms related to Th17 cells in allergy, autoimmunity, skin disease, nervous system, and carcinogenesis have been extended further in the last decades.

TH17 CELL IN ALLERGY

Allergic diseases have a high prevalence and include disorders such as atopic dermatitis/eczema, contact dermatitis, drug hypersensitivity, as well as allergic rhinitis, asthma, conjunctivitis, etc. Over an extended period, allergic diseases have been described as IgE-mediated disease where T-helper-2 (Th2) cells play a critical role [2]. After the discovery of new cytokines and T cells within the last years, it was shown that IL-17 and Th17 cells appear to be the fine-tuning regulator of the Th2-driven response in allergy [1].

The most crucial cytokine of Th17 cells, IL-17, is known to induce other pro-inflammatory cytokines (i.e., TNF-a, IL-1b, and IL-6), as well as chemokines CXCL1, 2, and 8, which attract neutrophils and other innate cells. In such way, IL-17 plays a crucial role in the initiation and maintaining the inflammatory processes [3-4].

As mentioned above, the neutrophil recruitment is a typical feature of Th17-mediated inflammation [2]. However, the role of Th17 cells in allergy is still mostly unclear, but experimental animal models suggest that Th17 cells control the extent of neutrophilic inflammation in acute airway inflammation [5].

Furthermore, neutrophils are responsible for the severe asthma attacks, where their increased number could be assessed in bronchoalveolar lavage. Interestingly, IL-17 mRNA levels in sputum correlate with CXCL8 and neutrophil counts in blood [2]. Furthermore, it is known that IL-17 contributes to the changes in human airway smooth muscles and airway epithelial cells through attraction of innate immune cells by chemoattractants [1, 2].

Acting together with other Th17-related cytokines, IL-17 induces the production of various mucous proteins to enhance inflammatory responses. In such a way, Th17 cells work by integrating the adaptive and innate immune mechanisms to provide protection. However, when uncontrolled, Th17-driven inflammation eventually leads to tissue damages. In contrast to the Th2-inflammation, where IFN-g enhances MHC-II expression in epithelial cells to become non-professional antigen-presenting cells or induces apoptosis in epithelial cells or keratinocytes, Th17-inflammation is fundamentally different.

Th17 cells, unlike Th2 cells, are capable of inducing metalloproteinases, which could be beneficial for reducing matrix deposition and avoiding remodeling of the airways [1].

Th17 cells also differ from Th1-driven inflammation because the former mediates tissue inflammation by stimulating neutrophil recruitment and survival, induction of pro-inflammatory cytokines, and matrix degradation.

Although almost all known functions of Th17 cells lead to inflammation and destruction, we have to keep in mind that this cell subtype also serves to protect the airways from bacteria and fungi in healthy individuals. In line with this, proper engagement of T regulatory cells could control the inflammation and redirects the processes towards immune homeostasis.

Th17 Cells in Autoimmune Skin Disease

Current knowledge on the role of Th17 cells and related cytokines in the pathogenesis of most blistering skin diseases, such as pemphigus vulgaris (PV) is limited. It is thought that many cytokines and chemokines take part – IFNg, RANTES, MCP-1, 2, 3, etc. [9].

More recently, it was shown that Th17 cells could also be involved in triggering and maintenance PV. However, Th17 cell expansion was dependent on the presence of IL-23 produced by macrophages and dendritic cells in injured tissues [7]. Patients with PV have increased serum levels of IFN-γ and IL-17; thus, both Th1 and Th17 subtypes are involved, which reinforces the observation that the immune responses in PV include a mix of Th1/Th17 immune mechanisms. It is assumed that higher levels of IL-23, together with IL-6, may enhance the production of IL-17 and promote Th17 differentiation, which probably contributed to the pathogenesis of PV [6]. However, most studies did not report elevated levels of IL-22, a cytokine produced by both Th17 and Th22 cells, suggesting that Th22 phenotype is not systemically induced in PV patients [8].

However, the positive association between skin lesions, Th1- and Th17- related cytokines and chemokines and disease activity in patients with PV, demonstrated by Timoteo et al. [6], supports the role of these immune responses in the pathogenesis of the disease.

Regarding the IL-17A levels in other blistering skin disorders, in a single study Zebrowska et al. demonstrated significantly higher expression of this cytokine in the perilesional epidermal skin biopsy and the serum of dermatitis herpetiformis (DH) and bullous pemphigoid patients, compared to the control group [9]. We also conducted a study in DH patients, where the results showed 60-fold higher concentrations of IL-17A in DH patients in comparison with healthy controls (p = 0.031) [10]. These two studies are amongst the few studies providing data for the involvement of IL-17 in DH and other blistering diseases pathogenesis.

Besides, Juczynska et al. reported increased expression of JAK/STAT proteins in skin lesions in patients with DH and bullous pemphigoid in comparison to perilesional skin and healthy controls [11]. The investigators also suggested that pro-inflammatory cytokine production, together with the inflammatory cell infiltrate in tissues contribute to the pathogenesis of skin lesions in both diseases. However, more studies are needed to establish the role of IL-17/Th17 cells in blistering skin diseases to tailor new therapeutic strategies based on new knowledge.

TH17 CELLS IN OTHER RHEUMATIC AUTOIMMUNE DISORDERS

Th17 cells are topic of discussion regarding their contribution to the pathogenesis of many autoimmune diseases such as multiple sclerosis (MS), rheumatoid arthritis (RA), systemic lupus erythematosus (SLE), psoriasis, systemic sclerosis (SSc), and inflammatory bowel disease (IBD) [12]. For example, serum and tissue/fluid samples (such as CSF from patients with MS, or synovial fluid in RA patients, etc.) exerted higher concentrations of IL-17 than healthy controls [13-15].

The role of Th17 cells in the pathogenesis of RA, MS, SSc, SLE, IBD has been demonstrated [12] first in animal models, then in patients. Our group also showed that IL-17 is present in elevated amounts in synovial fluid taken from the inflamed joints, in the peripheral blood in RA [16]. Besides, Th17 cells were at increased number and percentages in patients with RA, reinforcing the pathogenic nature of Th17 cells in RA, not only locally, but Th17 cells also contribute to systemic inflammation typical for the disease [17, 18]. Th17 roles in autoimmunity were initially observed in gastrointestinal autoimmune disorders, such as IBD patients, in whom both high percentages of peripheral blood Th17 cells and high IL-17A concentrations in the intestinal mucosa have been assessed [19-22]. On the contrary, Tregs were estimated at a low number and percentages, indicating the problem with controlling the pathological expansion of Th17 cells and the impaired Th17/Treg balance [20, 22]. It is essential to emphasize again that Tregs play a pivotal role in the prevention of these

Th17-mediated autoimmune diseases [6, 12]. Some of the therapies available on the market for autoimmune diseases, such as anti-TNFa drugs, may increase the numbers of Tregs, contributing this way to the alleviating of the symptoms and helping the healing of the affected tissues [23-29].

Changes in the balance between Tregs and Th17 cells have been implicated in shifting the balance between limiting and sustained autoimmunity [30]. Furthermore, the plasticity of Th17 cells contributes to a specific disease in a predominantly inflammatory milieu [30].

Several genes identified by GWAS were examined to find how the activity and plasticity of Th17 cells are influenced by TCR and cytokine signaling [23]. In addition to this various SNPs were associated with changes in gene expression levels and alteration in cytokine signaling proteins, which was directly linked to Th17 cell functions [23].

Other typical features of Th17 cells that contribute to the autoimmunity are the following: lower activation thresholds than Th1 cells, which make them more prone to become self-reactive effector cells [31]. Other factors are the environmental and bacterial antigens that after penetration of the mucosa exert persisting triggering of self-reactive Th17 responses in the gut [31, 32]. It was also shown that IL-23 and apoptotic epithelial cells favorably promoted self-reactive Th17 cells and autoantibody production [32]. This showed the link between the Th17 cells, B-cell activation, and autoantibody production, observed in many autoimmune diseases [23]. For example, the B-cell activating factor (BAFF), known as essential for B-cell activation and differentiation, also promotes Th17 differentiation by upregulation of the IL-6 receptor on CD4+ T cells [33].

Although many mechanisms related to Th17 involvement in autoimmunity are revealed, the majority of their effects remain unclear.

TH17 CELLS IN THE NERVOUS SYSTEM

Multiple sclerosis (MS) is one of the most common autoimmune diseases of the central nervous system (CNS). Several animal models of experimental autoimmune encephalomyelitis (EAE) have proven the autoimmune nature of the disease [34]. Today, it is known that Th17 cells contribute to the organ-specific autoimmune features of the EAE and MS as well as in their immunopathology. Moreover, here, the plasticity of the Th17 subset is shown once again, as well as their ability in promoting these debilitating diseases [34].

A recent study showed that human CD4+ T cells that exhibit Th17 phenotype have a higher capacity than Th1 differentiated cells to penetrate the blood brain barrier and infiltrate the parenchyma of the CNS [35]. It has been also demonstrated that endothelial cells of the human blood brain barrier decrease the expression of tight junction proteins when culturing with recombinant IL-17. This explains why Th17 cells can transmigrate in the CNS through the blood brain barrier, allowing migration of other inflammatory cells as well [34]. Other mechanisms that would enable Th17 cells to enter the blood brain barriers are expressing CCR6 and used the expressed CCR6 ligand CCL20 on epithelium of the choroid plexus to access the subarachnoid space and initiate inflammation [36]. This pattern of CNS infiltration by Th17 cells is mediated by the integrin LFA-1, whereas Th1 cells target the spinal cord in a VLA-4 dependent manner [34].

The pathological hallmarks of CNS autoimmunity are inflammation, demyelination, and axonal damage [34]. The breakdown of the blood brain barrier with subsequent infiltration of mononuclear cells is considered an essential prerequisite for the development of autoimmune inflammatory lesions in the CNS. The mechanism of action of Th17 cells in this destructive cascade has only partially been unraveled so far. It is assumed that together with IL-17, granulocyte macrophage-colony factor (GM-CSF), IL-9, IL-21, and IL-22 contribute to the CNS autoimmunity [34]. IL-17 can also stimulate epithelial cells to produce CXCL1 and CXCL2 that have been detected in lesions of patients with EAE and MS. Consequently, large numbers of leukocytes can be recruited to the perivascular white matter. Furthermore, IL-17 provokes excess oxidative stress in the endothelial cells leading eventually to an impaired barrier function [37]. There is also evidence that direct interactions of Th17 cells with neurons in

212   *Tsvetelina Velikova*

demyelinating lesions induce severe neuronal dysfunction [38], whereas the exact mechanism remains non-elucidated.

In conclusion, there is evidence for a wide range of proinflammatory and neurotoxic effects exerted by IL-17 in CNS autoimmunity. However, several studies indicated that IL-17 neutralizing is an excellent approach attenuate the EAE, although never reverse it [34]. The explanation for this is related to the fact that several factors play a role in CNS autoimmunity – except Th17 cells, Th1 cells, as well as many other cytokines, drive the pathology in the absence of IL-17.

A new novel study by Ribeiro et al. [39] showed that meningeal gd T cell-derived IL-17 controls synaptic plasticity and short-term memory. This can help to understand other beneficial roles of tTh17 cells, except its pathological functions of in CNS.

TH17 CELLS AND CARCINOGENESIS

Chronic inflammation, typical for IBD patients, is proven to be a risk factor for the development of colorectal cancer (CRC) [40]. Carcinogenesis is based on the mucosal injury following the intestinal inflammation, triggered long-lasting healing responses, tissue dysfunction, and increased cell turnover [41]. Th17 cells and their related cytokines are also involved in CRC developments in animals and humans. It was shown that Th17 cells were abundant in tumors of CRC patients, and increased Th17-related cytokines correlate with advanced stages of CRC [43-45].

However, in the context of CRC, Th17 cells should be distinguished from their signature cytokines, IL-17A. IL-17A in mouse IBD models exerted the protective function that can be explained by the effect of this cytokine on enterocytes. Similar to IL-22, IL-17A can induce their proliferation and can enhance tight-barrier formation. In this way, IL-17 promotes the integrity of the epithelial barrier [34]. On the other side, the same regenerative and physiological effects of IL-17A can promote carcinogenesis in the colon too. Also, bacterial translocation and IL-23 production by innate immune cells lead to the upregulation of IL-17A levels, which in turn can favor intestinal tumorigenesis [46]. It was further shown that the increased number of IL-17A producing cells found in human CRC and elevated IL-17 mRNA expression correlates with a poor prognosis in CRC patients [47-49]. Although these findings point to a potential therapeutic benefit of anti-IL-17A treatment, the heterogeneity of Th17 cells makes it impossible to conclude their exact function in human CRC, and further research is needed before initiating clinical trials [34].

Since the abundancy of Th17 cells in IBD and several genetic risk loci have linked between Th17 cells and IBD, some drugs were developed to manipulate Th17 cell development or function in patients with IBD. However, the results were controversial, even aggravated disease course in IBD patients was reported, which can be explained by the suppressed beneficial effects of IL-17 when targeted.

In contrast, Ustekinumab, a monoclonal antibody against IL-23, proved to be effective in preventing colitis in mouse models and patients with Crohn`s disease [50]. Anti-TNF therapy is already well established in the treatment of both forms of IBD.

Surprisingly, it was recently shown that the effectiveness of this therapy is, to some extent, dependent on the IL-22–IL-22BP axis in both mice and humans [51]. However, the oncogenic potential of IL-22 could represent a significant obstacle in the development of safe and drugs targeting this axis.

CONCLUSION

The role of Th17 cells in autoimmune, inflammatory, allergic, and tumor diseases has been reported and supported by some studies. Interestingly, Th17 cells exhibit similar behaviors in the conditions where Th17 cells are considered to play a role. Furthermore, the number of diseases influenced by Th17 cells appears to be increasing. However, in most of them, the exact mechanism of actions of Th17 cells remain unclear, though evidence suggests that they could also play an essential role in the control of these diseases.

REFERENCES

[1] Schmidt-Weber, C. B., Akdis, M., Akdis, C. A. TH17 cells in the big picture of immunology. *J. Allergy Clin. Immunol.*, 2007; 120(2):247 - 54.

[2] Hofmann, M. A., Kiecker, F., Zuberbier, T. A systematic review of the role of interleukin-17 and the interleukin-20 family in inflammatory allergic skin diseases. *Curr. Opin. Allergy Clin. Immunol.*, 2016; 16(5):451 - 7.

[3] Yao, Z., Painter, S. L., Fanslow, W. C., Ulrich, D., Macduff, B. M., Spriggs, M. K. et al. Human IL-17: a novel cytokine derived from T cells. *J. Immunol.*, 1995; 155:5483 - 6.

[4] Awane, M., Andres, P. G., Li, D. J., Reinecker, H. C. NF-kappa B-inducing kinase is a common mediator of IL-17-, TNF-alpha-, and IL-1 betainduced chemokine promoter activation in intestinal epithelial cells. *J. Immunol.*, 1999; 162:5337 - 44.

[5] Hashimoto, T., Akiyama, K., Kobayashi, N., Mori, A. Comparison of IL-17 production by helper T cells among atopic and nonatopic asthmatics and control subjects. *Int. Arch. Allergy Immunol.*, 2005; 137(suppl. 1):51 - 4.

[6] Timoteo, R. P., de Silva, M. V., Miguel, C. B. et al. Th1/Th17-Related Cytokines and Chemokines and Their Implications in the Pathogenesis of Pemphigus Vulgaris. *Mediators of Inflammation*, 2017; 2017, 7151285, 9 pages.

[7] Xue, J., Su, W., Chen, Z. et al. Overexpression of interleukin-23 and interleukin-17 in the lesion of pemphigus vulgaris: a preliminary study, *Mediators of Inflammation*, 2014; 2014, Article ID 463928, 5 pages.

[8] Mortazavi, H., Esmaili, N., Khezri, S. et al. The effect of conventional immunosuppressive therapy on cytokine serum levels in pemphigus vulgaris patients, *Iranian Journal of Allergy, Asthma and Immunology*, 2014; 13(3):174 - 183.

[9] Zebrowska, A., Wagrowska-Danilewicz, M., Danilewicz, M., Stasikowska-Kanicka, O., Cynkier, A., Sysa-Jedrzejowska, A.,

Waszczykowska, E. IL-17 Expression in Dermatitis Herpetiformis and Bullous Pemphigoid. *Mediat. Inflamm.*, 2013; 2013:967987.

[10] Velikova, T., Shahid, M., Ivanova-Todorova, E. et al. Celiac-Related Autoantibodies and IL-17A in Bulgarian Patients with Dermatitis Herpetiformis: A Cross-Sectional Study. *Medicina,* (Kaunas). 2019; 55(5):136.

[11] Juczynska, K., Wozniacka, A., Waszczykowska, E., Danilewicz, M., Wagrowska-Danilewicz, M., Wieczfinska, J., Pawliczak, R., Zebrowska, A. Expression of the JAK/STAT Signaling Pathway in Bullous Pemphigoid and Dermatitis Herpetiformis. *Mediat. Inflamm.*, 2017; 2017:6716419.

[12] Bystrom, J., Clanchy, F. I. L., Taher, T. E. et al. Functional and phenotypic heterogeneity of Th17 cells in health and disease. *Eur. J. Clin. Invest.,* 2019; 49:e13032.

[13] Jain, R., Chen, Y., Kanno, Y. et al. Interleukin-23-induced transcription factor Blimp-1 promotes pathogenicity of T helper 17 cells. *Immunity,* 2016; 44:131 - 142.

[14] Fang, Z., Hecklau, K., Gross, F. et al. Transcription factor co-occupied regions in the murine genome constitute T-helper-cell subtype-specific enhancers. *Eur. J. Immunol.,* 2015; 45:3150 - 3157.

[15] Gaublomme, J. T., Yosef, N., Lee, Y. et al. Single-cell genomics unveils critical regulators of Th17 cell pathogenicity. *Cell,* 2015; 163:1400 - 1412.

[16] Velikova, T., Shumnalieva, R., Kachakova, D. et al. IL-17A – A Promising Biomarker for Disease Activity in Rheumatoid Arthritis Patients. *Journal of Biomedical Science and Technology,* 2018; 1(1): 6 - 20.

[17] Kebir, H., Kreymborg, K., Ifergan, I. et al. Human TH17 lymphocytes promote blood-brain barrier disruption and central nervous system inflammation. *Nat. Med.,* 2007; 13:1173 - 1175.

[18] Evans, H. G., Roostalu, U., Walter, G. J. et al. TNF-alpha blockade induces IL-10 expression in human CD4 + T cells. *Nat. Commun.,* 2014; 5:3199.

[19] Velikova, Ts. *Investigation of immunological parameters for intestinal inflammation in order to establish new markers for diagnosis and follow-up of Inflammatory Bowel Disease patients.* Dissertation 2014. Medical University of Sofia.

[20] Velikova, T., Kyurkchiev, D., Spassova, Z. et al. Alterations in cytokine gene expression profile in colon mucosa of Inflammatory Bowel Disease patients on different therapeutic regimens. *Cytokine,* 2017; 92:12 - 19.

[21] Eastaff-Leung, N. *Regulatory T Cells, Th17 Effector cells and cytokine microenvironment in inflammatory bowel disease and coeliac disease*; 2009.Dissertation.

[22] Eastaff-Leung, N., Mabarrack, N., Barbour, A., Cummins, A., Barry, S. Foxp3+ regulatory T cells, Th17 effector cells, and cytokine environment in inflammatory bowel disease. *Journal of clinical immunology,* 2010; 30(1):80 - 89.

[23] Bystrom, J., Clanchy, F. I., Taher, T. E. et al. TNFa in the regulation of Treg and Th17 cells in rheumatoid arthritis and other autoimmune inflammatory diseases. *Cytokine,* 2016; 101:4 - 13.

[24] Boschetti, G., Nancey, S., Sardi, F. Therapy with anti-TNFα antibody enhances number and function of Foxp3(+) regulatory T cells in inflammatory bowel diseases. *Inflamm. Bowel Dis.,* 2011; 17(1):160 - 70.

[25] Heetun, Z., Doherty, G. A. Restoring the Regulatory Regime in IBD: Do Anti-TNF Agents Rescue Treg? *Inflammatory Bowel Diseases,* 2012, 18(6):1186 - 1187.

[26] Veltkamp, C., Anstaett, M., Wahl, K. et al. Apoptosis of regulatory T lymphocytes is increased in chronic inflammatory bowel disease and reversed by anti-TNFα treatment. *Gut,* 2011; 60(10):1345 - 53.

[27] Guidi, L., Felice, C., Procoli, A. et al. FOXP3+ T Regulatory Cell Modifications in Inflammatory Bowel Disease Patients Treated with Anti-TNF Agents. *Bio. Med. Research International,* 2013; 2013, Article ID 286368, 10 pages.

[28] Liu, C., Xia, X., Wu, W. et al. Anti-tumour necrosis factor therapy enhances mucosal healing through down-regulation of interleukin-21

expression and T helper type 17 cell infiltration in Crohn's disease. *Clin. Exp. Immunol.*, 2013; 173(1):102 - 11.

[29] Ueno, A., Jijon, H., Chan, R. et al. Increased prevalence of circulating novel IL-17 secreting Foxp3 expressing CD4+ T cells and defective suppressive function of circulating Foxp3+ regulatory cells support plasticity between Th17 and regulatory T cells in inflammatory bowel disease patients. *Inflamm. Bowel Dis.*, 2013; 19(12):2522 - 34.

[30] McGovern, J. L., Nguyen, D. X., Notley, C. A., Mauri, C., Isenberg, D. A., Ehrenstein, M. R. Th17 cells are restrained by Treg cells via the inhibition of interleukin-6 in patients with rheumatoid arthritis responding to anti-tumor necrosis factor antibody therapy. *Arthritis Rheum.*, 2012; 64:3129 - 3138.

[31] Purvis, H. A., Stoop, J. N., Mann, J. et al. Low-strength T-cell activation promotes Th17 responses. *Blood*, 2010; 116:4829 - 4837.

[32] Atarashi, K., Tanoue, T., Ando, M. et al. Th17 cell induction by adhesion of microbes to intestinal epithelial cells. *Cell*, 2015; 163:367 - 380.

[33] Zhou, X., Xia, Z., Lan, Q. et al. BAFF promotes Th17 cells and aggravates experimental autoimmune encephalomyelitis. *PLoS ONE*, 2011; 6:e23629.

[34] Sie, C., Korn, T., Mitsdoerffer, M. Th17 cells in central nervous system autoimmunity. *Exp. Neurol.*, 2014; 262 Pt A:18 - 27.

[35] Zielinski, C. E., Mele, F., Aschenbrenner, D. et al. Pathogen-induced human TH17 cells produce IFN-gamma or IL-10 and are regulated by IL-1beta. *Nature*, 2012; 484:514 - 518.

[36] Reboldi, A., Coisne, C., Baumjohann, D. et al. C–C chemokine receptor 6-regulated entry of TH-17 cells into the CNS through the choroid plexus is required for the initiation of EAE. *Nat. Immunol.*, 10, 514 - 523.

[37] Huppert, J., Closhen, D., Croxford, A. et al. Cellular mechanisms of IL-17-induced blood–brain barrier disruption. *FASEB J.*, 2010; 24, 1023 - 1034.

[38] Siffrin, V., Radbruch, H., Glumm, R. et al. In vivo imaging of partially reversible th17 cell-induced neuronal dysfunction in the course of encephalomyelitis. *Immunity,* 2010; 33, 424 - 436.

[39] Ribeiro, M., Brigas, H., Temido-Ferreira, M. et al. Meningeal γδ T cell–derived IL-17 controls synaptic plasticity and short-term memory. *Science Immunology*, 2019:4(40):eaay5199.

[40] Kempski, J., Brockmann, L., Gagliani, N., Huber, S. TH17 Cell and Epithelial Cell Crosstalk during Inflammatory Bowel Disease and Carcinogenesis. *Front. Immunol.,* 2017; 8:1373.

[41] Antonio, N., Bonnelykke-Behrndtz, M. L., Ward, L. C., Collin, J., Christensen, I. J., Steiniche, T. et al. The wound inflammatory response exacerbates growth of pre-neoplastic cells and progression to cancer. *EMBO J.,* (2015) 34(17):2219 - 36.

[42] Stanilov, N., Miteva, L., Girovski, G., Stanilova, S. Upregulation of Treg and downregulation of Th17 related cytokine expression in peripheral blood of colorectal cancer patients. *Trakia Journal of Sciences,* 2014; 12(1):150 - 156.

[43] Amicarella, F., Muraro, M. G., Hirt, C. et al. Dual role of tumour-infiltrating T helper 17 cells in human colorectal cancer. *Gut,* 2017; 66(4):692 - 704.

[44] Mao, H., Pan, F., Guo, H. et al. Feedback mechanisms between M2 macrophages and Th17 cells in colorectal cancer patients. *Tumour Biol.*, 2016; 37(9):12223 - 30.

[45] Sharp, S. P., Avram, D., Stain, S. C., Lee, E. C. Local and systemic Th17 immune response associated with advanced stage colon cancer. *J. Surg. Res.,* 2017; 208:180 - 6.

[46] Grivennikov, S. I., Wang, K., Mucida, D., Stewart, C. A., Schnabl, B., Jauch, D. et al. Adenoma-linked barrier defects and microbial products drive IL-23/IL-17- mediated tumour growth. *Nature,* (2012) 491(7423):254 - 8.

[47] Wang, K., Kim, M. K., Di Caro, G., Wong, J., Shalapour, S., Wan, J. et al. Interleukin-17 receptor a signaling in transformed enterocytes promotes early colorectal tumorigenesis. *Immunity,* 2014; 41(6): 1052 - 63.

[48] Dunne, M. R., Ryan, C., Nolan, B., Tosetto, M., Geraghty, R., Winter, D. C. et al. Enrichment of inflammatory IL-17 and TNF-alpha secreting CD4(+) T cells within colorectal tumors despite the presence of elevated CD39(+) T regulatory cells and increased expression of the immune checkpoint molecule, PD-1. *Front. Oncol.,* 2016; 6:50.

[49] Mlecnik, B., Bindea, G., Angell, H. K., Maby, P., Angelova, M., Tougeron, D. et al. Integrative analyses of colorectal cancer show immunoscore is a stronger predictor of patient survival than microsatellite instability. *Immunity,* (2016) 44(3):698 - 711.

[50] Feagan, B. G., Sandborn, W. J., Gasink, C. et al. Ustekinumab as induction and maintenance therapy for Crohn's disease. *N Engl. J. Med.,* 2016; 375(20):1946 - 60.

[51] Pelczar, P., Witkowski, M., Perez, L. G., Kempski, J., Hammel, A. G., Brockmann, L. et al. A pathogenic role for T cell-derived IL-22BP in inflammatory bowel disease. *Science,* (2016) 354 (6310): 358 - 62.

In: Th17 Cells in Health and Disease
Editor: Tsvetelina Velikova

ISBN: 978-1-53617-152-5
© 2020 Nova Science Publishers, Inc.

Chapter 13

THE CONTROVERSIAL INTERACTION BETWEEN TH17 AND T REGULATORY CELLS IN AUTOIMMUNITY

Tsvetelina Velikova[*], MD, PhD
Clinical Immunology, University Hospital Lozenetz,
Medical Faculty, Sofia University, Sofia, Bulgaria

ABSTRACT

Th17 lymphocytes play a role both in protecting the organism from infectious agents and in the pathogenesis of several autoimmune diseases. Regulatory CD4+CD25+/-FoxP3+ lymphocytes (Treg) follow a different pathway of differentiation compare to Th17 lymphocytes. However, the balance between the two subpopulations is the basis for preservation of immunologic homeostasis in the body.

The balance between Th17 and Treg is critical for immune homeostasis in the body, especially for preventing autoimmune diseases. Typically, the functions of Treg and Th17 cells must be reciprocally balanced, where changes in the cytokine environment may lead to polarization and dominance of one or another type of effector immune

---

[*] Corresponding Author's Email: tsvelikova@medfac.mu-sofia.bg.

response - inflammation or tolerance. Studies confirm that Treg cells isolated from the inflamed tissues are functionally suppressed ex vivo, suggesting their inability to inhibit Th17 responses in the organism, especially in an environment rich in pro-inflammatory cytokines, such as the ambiguous IL-6. This gives hope that suppression of the activity of IL-6 can affect the balance between Th17 and Treg and alleviate autoimmune symptoms. Moreover, the described conversion between Th17 and Treg makes the picture more complicated and confusing. Regulation of this balance, as well as the control of Th17-mediated inflammation, are the main elements in the development of therapeutic strategies for some autoimmune diseases.

Keywords: Th17 cells, T regulatory cells, Tregs, TGFb, IL-17, IL-6

INTRODUCTION

Speaking of T lymphocytes, it is known that in addition to inflammatory effector cells (CD4+, different types of T-helper cells), there are also regulatory subpopulations. It is understood that the immunological homeostasis depends on the balance between effector and regulatory responses [1].

Th17 cells are key players in many pathological processes in humans and animal models. Fujino et al. were the first to identify Th17 cells as a significant source of IL-17 in patients with Inflammatory Bowel Disease (IBD) in 2003 [2]. They were the first also to describe the significantly higher levels of IL-17 in the serum of patients with IBD compared to healthy subjects [2]. Thus, Th17 lymphocytes and cytokines related to their development and maintenance (IL-6, TGFβ1, IL-23, and others) represent a distinctive immunological feature of immune response, outlining a novel, different route of interaction between innate and acquired mechanisms of immunity [3].

In our previous studies, we investigate the role of the proinflammatory Th17 and CD4+ CD25+FoxP3+ T regulatory cells (Treg) locally in the inflamed intestinal mucosa in IBD patients and followed-up their interactions [1].

Th17 vs. Treg Cells in Health and Disease

Our results on Th17 vs. Treg cells showed that the gene expression of FoxP3, IL-10, IL-17A, IL-23, IL-6, and TGFβ1 was higher in patients with IBD compared to healthy controls. Furthermore, in most IBD patients the expression of the markers mentioned above was significantly higher in the affected intestinal tissue, than the adjacent healthy tissue. Genes for TGFβ1 were expressed in the majority of patients, and IL-17A genes were expressed in the fewest patients. Thus, the expression of the genes we study was sorted in the order from the strongest expression to the least expressed: TGFβ1, FoxP3, IL-10, IL-23, IL-6, IL-17A [4].

Regarding the control group of healthy subjects, expression of TGFβ1, FoxP3, and IL-10 was observed in all subjects, while the remaining genes for IL-23, IL-17A, and IL-6 were expressed only in a limited number of individuals. We demonstrated the dominant presence of suppressive cytokines IL-10 and TGFβ1 in individuals without IBD, as well as the FoxP3 transcription factor as indirect marker for Tregs present [1, 4].

Even endoscopically distinguished, the normal mucosa of IBD patients exerted some genetic alterations, which suggested that these patients have a genetic ground for the development of the disease. Comparing the gene expression of cytokine levels in the inflamed mucosa of patients with IBD and those of the control group without IBD, we found about 5-fold higher levels of IL-17A mRNA expression in patients with IBD (RQ = 5.69). However, these results did not reach statistical significance, probably because of the limited number of patients who expressed the IL-17A gene [1]. Our results for IL-17A are in one way with those of Fonseca-Camarillo et al. and Eastaff-Leung et al., who also found increased expression of the IL-17A gene in inflamed mucosa of IBD patients [5-7].

However, all the factors necessary for Th17 lymphocyte differentiation in humans are not yet fully elucidated. There is evidence that IL-1b and IL-6 are required for differentiation of Th17 from memory T cells, whereas IL-21 and TGFβ1 are likely involved in Th17 differentiation from naïve T cells [5, 8]. According to most data in the literature, TGFβ1 is engaged in the development of reciprocal differentiation of both Th17 and Treg, possibly involving other cytokines [5].

We found significantly increased gene expression of both IL-6 and TGFβ1 cytokines in inflammatory tissue, i.e., our data supports the thesis of differentiation of naïve T cells in the proinflammatory effector subpopulation Th17. In favor of this hypothesis, we also found increased gene expression of IL-17A in patients with IBD [4].

On the other hand, we also obtained data on the involvement of Treg cells in the inflamed mucosa by a significantly increased expression of the FoxP3 transcription factor expressed constitutively by Tregs [1]. We have also found in the literature publications describing the high expression of FoxP3 in the mucosa and the peripheral blood of patients with IBD, i.e., secondary data for the presence of Tregs. However, Tregs themselves can be both CD4+ and recently described CD8+FoxP3+ Tregs [5], but we did not distinguish them. Based on our results for the FoxP3 transcription factor, we cannot determine whether the T regulatory cells are CD4 + or CD8 + lymphocytes.

Similar to our data on the simultaneous presence of reciprocal Th17 and Tregs cells in their differentiation and function have been found by other authors [5, 6]. One explanation for this is the active differentiation of Treg lymphocytes in the mucosa to suppress proinflammatory responses [6]. Another possible answer is that Treg cells in the mucosa of patients with IBD are not fully functional due to the presence of IL-6 [9]. Studies confirm that Treg isolated from the mucosa of patients with IBD are functionally suppressed ex vivo. This also implies their inability to inhibit Th17 responses in the mucosa, especially in an environment rich in proinflammatory cytokines [9]. Moreover, in the presence of IL-1β and IL-6, Treg can not only be suppressed but also are able to undergo conversion to Th17 cells [10] and thus promote disease progression.

Typically, the functions of Treg and Th17 cells must be balanced with each other, but changes in the cytokine environment of the mucosa may lead to reciprocal polarization and dominance of one or the other type of effector immune response - inflammation or tolerance. We believe that in our patients with IBD, the significantly higher gene expression of the

FoxP3 transcription factor suggests a proliferation of Tregs in the mucosa in an attempt to suppress pathological Th17 subpopulation, but elevated IL-6 renders them to exert they anti-inflammatory and regulatory properties [1]. In the last two years, IL-17 secreting Treg cells have also been described, which introduces controversy rather than light into the pathogenesis of IBD [10-13].

Taking into account that the terminally differentiated Th17 cells and Tregs fulfill opposite functions, it is essential to keep the balance between them to maintain the immunological homeostasis [14]. This is especially valid in autoimmunity, where Th17 cells contribute to autoimmune responses and inflammation, whereas Treg cells aim to suppress these phenomena and maintain immune homeostasis.

Regulation of Th17 cells by other CD4+, Treg cells, was first identified in 2001 [15]. After this, Tregs have been shown as critical to maintaining tolerance, including to prevent autoimmunity and allergy [16,17]. However, Tregs are not homogeneous group of cells, several subgroups are described, including natural (nTregs) that originate from the thymus and induced (iTregs), which are located in the peripheral lymphoid tissues [18].

Failure to regulate the cytokine environmental milieu and signaling potentially leads to an imbalance of different subsets of T-helper cells and subsequent development of inflammatory conditions. This is not surprising because the differentiation of CD4-naive T cell precursors to effector T helper cells depends on a large extent of the cytokine signals they receive in tissue environment [19]. In line with this, the essential role for the prevention of Th17-mediated autoimmune diseases is appointed to Tregs [19, 20].

In the context of autoimmunity, Tregs have two mechanisms through which they can exert their suppressive function. The first is by a cell–cell contact, which leads to release of IL-35 and inhibition of proliferation of pathogenic Th17 cells [20, 22, 23]. For example, patients with RA, IBD, and other autoimmune disorders, for which anti-TNFa therapy is approved, have increased numbers of Tregs [24-26]. It is thought that these stimulated Tregs can suppress pathogenic Th17 responses. Similarly, anti-

TNF-a treatment of patients with IBD results in increased peripheral Treg expression. Other studies have also demonstrated suppression of Th17 responses by Tregs in terms of numbers and cytokine production [20, 27].

CONCLUSION

In conclusion, shedding light on the mechanisms that control the Th17/Treg cell balance is critical for better understanding of autoimmunity and tolerance. Recent studies have identified many factors that influence this balance: cytokines, signaling pathways triggered by T cell receptors, costimulatory receptors, metabolic pathways, and the intestinal microbiota. Moreover, the described conversion between Th17 and Treg makes the picture more complicated and confusing. Regulation of this balance, as well as the control of Th17-mediated inflammation, are the main elements in the development of therapeutic strategies for some autoimmune diseases.

REFERENCES

[1] Velikova Ts. Investigation of immunological parameters for intestinal inflammation in order to establish new markers for diagnosis and follow-up of Inflammatory Bowel Disease patients. *Dissertation* 2014. Medical University of Sofia.

[2] Fujino S, Andoh A, Bamba S, Ogawa A, Hata K, Araki Y, et al. Increased expression of interleukin 17 in inflammatory bowel disease. *Gut*. 2003;52(1):65-70.

[3] Hundorfean G, Neurath MF, Mudter J. Functional relevance of T helper 17 (Th17) cells and the IL-17 cytokine family in inflammatory bowel disease. *Inflammatory Bowel Diseases*. 2011;18(1):180-186.

[4] Velikova T, Kyurkchiev D, Spassova Z, et al. Alterations in cytokine gene expression profile in colon mucosa of Inflammatory Bowel

Disease patients on different therapeutic regimens. *Cytokine.* 2017;92:12-19.

[5] Eastaff-Leung N. Regulatory T Cells, Th17 Effector cells and cytokine microenvironment in inflammatory bowel disease and coeliac disease; 2009. *Dissertation.*

[6] Eastaff-Leung N, Mabarrack N, Barbour A, Cummins A, Barry S. Foxp3+ regulatory T cells, Th17 effector cells, and cytokine environment in inflammatory bowel disease. *Journal of Clinical Immunology.* 2010;30(1):80-89.

[7] Fonseca-Camarillo G, Furuzawa-Carballeda J, Llorente L, Yamamoto-Furusho JK. IL-10-- and IL-20--expressing epithelial and inflammatory cells are increased in patients with ulcerative colitis. *Journal of Clinical Immunology.* 2011;33(3):640-648.

[8] Yang Y, Xu J, Niu Y, Bromberg JS, Ding Y. T-bet and eomesodermin play critical roles in directing T cell differentiation to Th1 versus Th17. *J. Immunol.* 2008;181(12):8700-8710.

[9] Maul J, Loddenkemper C, Mundt P, Berg E, Giese T, Stallmach A, et al. Peripheral and intestinal regulatory CD4+ CD25(high) T cells in inflammatory bowel disease. *Gastroenterology.* 2005;128(7):1868-1878.

[10] Koenen HJ, Smeets RL, Vink PM, van Rijssen E, Boots AM, Joosten I. Human CD25highFoxp3pos regulatory T cells differentiate into IL-17-producing cells. *Blood.* 2008;112(6):2340-2352.

[11] Beriou G, Costantino CM, Ashley CW, Yang L, Kuchroo VK, Baecher-Allan C, et al. IL-17-producing human peripheral regulatory T cells retain suppressive function. *Blood.* 2009;113(18):4240-4249.

[12] Kui Shin Vooa, Yui-Hsi Wanga, Fabio R. Santorib, Cesar Boggianob, Yi-Hong Wanga, Kazuhiko Arimaa, et al. Identification of IL-17-producing FOXP3+ regulatory T cells in humans. *PNAS.* 2009;106(12):4793-4798.

[13] Li L, Boussiotis V. The role of IL-17-producing Foxp3+ CD4+ T cells in inflammatory bowel disease and colon cancer. *Clin. Immunol.* 2013;148(2):246-253.

[14] Lee GR. The Balance of Th17 versus Treg Cells in Autoimmunity. *Int. J. Mol. Sci.* 2018;19(3):730.

[15] Bettelli E, Carrier Y, Gao W, et al. Reciprocal developmental pathways for the generation of pathogenic effector TH17 and regulatory T cells. *Nature* 2006;441: 235-38.

[16] Buckner JH. Mechanisms of impaired regulation by CD4(+)CD25(+)FOXP3(+) regulatory T cells in human autoimmune diseases. *Nat. Rev. Immunol.* 2010;10: 849-59.

[17] Carrier Y, Yuan J, Kuchroo VK, Weiner HL. Th3 cells in peripheral tolerance. II. TGF-beta-transgenic Th3 cells rescue IL-2-deficient mice from autoimmunity. *J. Immunol.* 2007;178: 172-8.

[18] Campbell DJ, Koch MA. Phenotypical and functional specialization of FOXP3+ regulatory T cells. *Nat. Rev. Immunol.* 2011;11: 119-30.

[19] Crome SQ, Clive B, Wang AY, et al. Inflammatory effects of *ex vivo* human Th17 cells are suppressed by regulatory T cells. *J. Immunol.* 2010; 185: 3199-208.

[20] Mondal S, Martinson JA, Ghosh S, et al. Protection of Tregs, suppression of Th1 and Th17 cells, and amelioration of experimental allergic encephalomyelitis by a physically-modified saline. *PLoS ONE* 2012;7: e51869.

[21] Gol-Ara M, Jadidi-Niaragh F, Sadria R, et al. The role of different subsets of regulatory T cells in immunopathogenesis of rheumatoid arthritis. *Arthritis* 2012: 805875.

[22] Josefowicz SZ, Lu LF, Rudensky AY. Regulatory T cells: mechanisms of differentiation and function. *Annu. Rev. Immunol.* 2012;30: 531-64.

[23] Niedbala W, Wei XQ, Cai B, et al. IL-35 is a novel cytokine with therapeutic effects against collagen-induced arthritis through the expansion of regulatory T cells and suppression of Th17 cells. *Eur. J. Immunol.* 2007;37: 3021-9.

[24] McGovern JL, Nguyen DX, Notley CA, et al. Th17 cells are restrained by Treg cells via the inhibition of interleukin-6 in patients with rheumatoid arthritis responding to anti-tumor necrosis factor antibody therapy. *Arthritis Rheum.* 2012;64: 3129-38.

[25] Bystrom J, Clanchy FI, Taher TE et al., TNFa in the regulation of Treg and Th17 cells in rheumatoid arthritis and other autoimmune inflammatory diseases. *Cytokine* 2016;101:4-13.

[26] Boschetti G, Nancey S, Sardi F. Therapy with anti-TNFα antibody enhances number and function of Foxp3(+) regulatory T cells in inflammatory bowel diseases. *Inflamm. Bowel Dis.* 2011;17(1):160-70.

[27] Fletcher JM, Lalor SJ, Sweeney CM, et al. T cells in multiple sclerosis and experimental autoimmune encephalomyelitis. *Clin. Exp. Immunol.* 2010;162: 1-11.

ABOUT THE EDITOR

Tsvetelina Veselinova Velikova
Assistant professor
Department of Clinical Immunology, Medical Faculty,
Sofia University, Sofia, Bulgaria
Email: tsvelikova@medfac.mu-sofia.bg

Dr. Tsvetelina Velikova received her MD and PhD degrees, both with honors, from the Medical University of Sofia, Bulgaria. Subsequently, she became involved in active immunology research and teaching. Dr. Velikova received also advanced training in Clinical immunology. She is currently an assistant professor of Clinical immunology affiliated to the Sofia University and University Hospital Lozenetz, Bulgaria. Her research focuses on autoimmune disorders and fine autoimmunity mechanisms involving Th17 and Treg cells, cytokines, biomarkers, novel biologic therapies and their implication in clinical practice. Dr. Velikova has been engaged in eighteen projects in the field of immunology and internal medicine. She is an editorial board member and reviewer for several medical journals and has publications in eminent journals and book chapters in the field of gastrointestinal immunology.

INDEX

A

acid, 39, 41, 43, 56, 104, 159, 174, 190
acquired immunity, 107, 157, 173
Adalimumab, 71, 80, 175, 176
adaptive immune responses, 35, 43, 59, 74, 130
adaptive immunity, 33, 35, 106, 120, 201
adhesion, 47, 69, 123, 126, 142, 143, 217
adolescents, 162, 165, 166
adults, 9, 100, 122, 153, 158, 192, 193, 195, 203
adverse effects, 123, 199
age, 4, 100, 101, 109, 117, 120, 153, 155, 156, 167, 176, 188, 198
air pollution, 84
airway hyperresponsiveness, 59
airway inflammation, 88, 99, 104, 106, 108, 109, 116, 121, 127, 128, 207
airway obstruction, 99, 100, 108
airway remodeling, 101, 108
airways, 83, 85, 86, 87, 92, 102, 110, 115, 117, 119, 121, 127, 128, 207
allergens, 85, 86, 91, 95, 100, 103
allergic asthma, 59, 101, 104, 110, 112, 113
allergic bronchopulmonary aspergillosis, 119, 130

allergic diseases, 84, 85, 89, 91, 93, 101, 102, 104, 105, 111, 131, 206
allergic inflammation, 85, 86, 87, 89, 90, 91, 96, 105, 113
allergic reactions, 87, 89, 121
allergic rhinitis, 83, 84, 85, 88, 90, 91, 93, 94, 95, 96, 97, 103, 104, 105, 106, 113, 206
allergy, 55, 59, 84, 86, 93, 94, 95, 96, 97, 107, 109, 110, 111, 112, 113, 129, 130, 131, 132, 205, 206, 207, 214, 225
angiogenesis, 13, 33, 62
ankylosing spondylitis, 54, 62, 72, 73, 74, 75, 76, 77, 78, 161
antibody, 9, 13, 14, 18, 19, 20, 22, 24, 27, 28, 43, 46, 65, 70, 72, 117, 118, 129, 185, 200, 216, 217, 228, 229
anti-DGP, 188, 190, 191, 193, 194, 198
antigen, 5, 34, 35, 41, 58, 62, 68, 70, 87, 89, 95, 119, 141, 143, 190, 191, 207
antigen-presenting cells, 35, 89, 95, 141, 143, 190, 191, 207
anti-IL-17 antibodies, 14, 17, 19, 20, 90
anti-TNF therapy, 71, 213
anti-TNFα therapy, 172, 174, 175, 176, 177, 179, 180, 181, 182, 183

234 *Index*

anti-tTG, 188, 193, 194, 196, 197, 198, 200, 203
apoptosis, 25, 102, 110, 125, 183, 207
apremilast, 68
arthralgia, 17, 26, 161
arthritis, 8, 11, 12, 13, 15, 19, 20, 21, 22, 23, 24, 25, 26, 27, 28, 45, 46, 47, 48, 49, 50, 51, 52, 57, 58, 59, 61, 62, 68, 71, 73, 74, 75, 76, 77, 78, 79, 80, 81, 111, 161, 217, 228
asthma, 59, 84, 86, 92, 93, 94, 96, 97, 99, 100, 101, 102, 103, 104, 105, 106, 107, 108, 109, 110, 111, 112, 113, 114, 123, 130, 131, 132, 206, 207, 214
autoantibodies, 32, 33, 40, 191, 192, 193, 194, 196, 203, 215
autoimmune disease, 6, 7, 17, 26, 32, 33, 35, 39, 45, 50, 52, 53, 58, 88, 138, 139, 141, 174, 187, 188, 194, 196, 209, 210, 221, 225, 226, 228
autoimmune diseases, 6, 7, 17, 33, 35, 39, 50, 52, 53, 88, 141, 174, 188, 194, 196, 209, 210, 221, 225, 226, 228
autoimmune skin disease, 208
autoimmunity, 32, 36, 37, 38, 39, 42, 46, 48, 50, 52, 57, 58, 101, 112, 205, 206, 209, 210, 211, 212, 217, 221, 225, 226, 228, 231
autonomic nervous system, 198
autosomal recessive, 115, 116
axial SpA, 62
axonal degeneration, 138
Azathioprine, 176, 195
azithromycin, 123, 124, 125, 126, 132, 133, 134, 135, 136

B

bacteria, 1, 4, 39, 58, 86, 107, 118, 122, 125, 158, 207
bacterial infection, 5, 39, 107, 117, 123

behaviors, 35, 44, 205, 213
beneficial effect, 123, 126, 213
biological activities, 41, 111
biological therapy, 172, 174, 184
biomarkers, 79, 162, 231
biopsy, 36, 92, 102, 166, 194, 208
blistering skin diseases, 206, 208, 209
blood, 7, 23, 42, 44, 46, 53, 54, 138, 140, 141, 142, 143, 144, 146, 161, 170, 182, 198, 207, 209, 211, 215, 217
blood-brain barrier, 138, 140, 142, 143, 146, 211
bone, 11, 12, 13, 14, 15, 16, 19, 20, 21, 22, 23, 24, 63, 64, 65, 66, 67, 68, 69, 71, 72, 74, 76, 77, 78, 79, 81, 195
bone destruction, 11, 12, 13, 14, 15, 16, 19, 21, 22, 66, 67, 69, 72
bone form, 65, 66, 67, 69, 72, 77, 78
bone formation, 65, 66, 67, 69, 72, 77, 78
bone marrow, 13, 14, 23, 65, 76, 79
bone resorption, 22, 24, 67, 72
bowel, 151, 153, 154, 162, 165, 166, 167, 168, 169, 172, 201
brain, 111, 138, 140, 141, 142, 143, 146, 198, 211, 215, 217
Brodalumab, 72
bronchial asthma, 84, 86, 92, 96, 97, 99, 101, 103, 105, 106, 107, 108, 109, 113
bronchial hyperreactivity, 86, 91, 99, 100, 101, 103, 106
bronchial hyperresponsiveness, 87, 96
bronchial mucosa, 92, 130
bronchiectasis, 116, 123, 132
bronchiolitis obliterans syndrome, 134
broncho-alveolar lavage, 102
bullous pemphigoid, 208

C

cancer, 57, 212, 218, 219
cancerogenesis, 206

Index

Candida albicans, 3

carcinogenesis, 205, 206, 212, 218

cartilage destruction, 14

CCR6, 14, 23, 39, 50, 52, 71, 144, 159, 169, 177, 211

CD4+ T lymphocytes, 2, 91, 177, 183

CD8+ T, 40, 62, 69, 70, 73, 75, 79, 103, 140, 144, 191

celiac disease, 187, 188, 189, 190, 196, 199, 200, 201, 202, 203, 204

cell differentiation, 3, 27, 39, 41, 55, 56

central nervous system, 138, 144, 147, 210, 215, 217

chemokine receptor, 25, 133, 141, 159, 217

chemokines, 15, 23, 25, 38, 39, 47, 68, 88, 104, 105, 107, 112, 124, 133, 134, 141, 142, 143, 159, 206, 208, 214, 217

childhood, 100, 101, 102, 108, 109, 111, 153, 154, 155, 156, 157, 160, 161, 163, 167, 169, 202

childhood asthma, 99, 100, 101, 102, 108, 109, 111

children, 4, 5, 9, 99, 100, 104, 105, 106, 108, 109, 112, 114, 120, 128, 130, 131, 132, 147, 148, 152, 153, 155, 156, 158, 159, 160, 162, 165, 166, 167, 170, 192, 193, 195

chronic infection, 118, 121, 125

chronic obstructive pulmonary disease, 100, 108, 109, 134

classification, 110, 153, 162, 163, 166, 170, 184

clinical presentation, 102, 163, 164, 166, 192

clinical symptoms, 90, 91, 190, 192, 195

clinical trials, 2, 5, 7, 126, 199, 213

clinically isolated syndrome, 143, 144, 148

colitis, 111, 112, 155, 162, 163, 164, 165, 166, 194, 213

collagen, 13, 15, 24, 28, 31, 32, 33, 37, 38, 40, 42, 44, 49, 51, 124, 228

colon, 2, 153, 155, 163, 172, 185, 212, 216, 218, 226, 227

colon cancer, 218, 227

colonization, 4, 5, 117, 123

colorectal cancer, 212, 218, 219

complications, 151, 154, 165, 173, 188, 197, 198

composition, 58, 185

conductance, 116, 129

conjunctivitis, 161, 206

connective tissue, 31, 32, 42, 57

consensus, 161, 166, 184

control group, 208, 223

controversies, 166, 184

correlation, 28, 42, 47, 86, 90, 91, 92, 120, 121, 144

corticosteroid resistant airway inflammation, 116, 121

corticosteroids, 103, 104, 105

Crohn's Disease (CD), 142, 152, 153, 154, 155, 156, 157, 158, 160, 161, 162, 163, 172, 182

CSF, 2, 14, 15, 37, 63, 71, 87, 103, 126, 142, 144, 209, 211

cystic fibrosis, 103, 107, 115, 116, 117, 118, 119, 120, 121, 122, 123, 125, 126, 127, 128, 129, 130, 131, 132, 133, 135, 136

cytotoxic lymphocyte antigen 8, 62

D

dactylitis, 61, 69, 70

damages, 139, 143, 207

deficiencies, 41, 192

deficiency, 42, 44, 90, 119, 131, 139, 158, 161, 193, 195, 196

demyelinating disease, 138, 147

demyelination, 138, 139, 143, 211

dendritic cells, 34, 39, 40, 43, 52, 57, 58, 69, 87, 105, 141, 142, 208

deposition, 31, 32, 33, 43, 51, 124, 197, 207

236 *Index*

dermal fibrosis, 36, 37
dermal vascular smooth muscle cells, 38, 42, 51
destruction, 11, 12, 13, 14, 15, 16, 19, 21, 22, 23, 66, 67, 69, 72, 142, 207
detection, 17, 175, 196
diet, 188, 189, 190, 193, 194, 195, 196, 198
disability, 42, 57, 138, 139
disease activity, 18, 28, 37, 38, 47, 49, 50, 54, 57, 64, 70, 71, 78, 141, 144, 148, 162, 170, 208
disease progression, 117, 154, 195, 197, 224
diseases, 4, 7, 33, 35, 42, 57, 84, 85, 88, 89, 91, 92, 93, 95, 100, 101, 102, 103, 104, 105, 106, 111, 124, 139, 156, 165, 168, 169, 172, 194, 196, 197, 205, 206, 208, 209, 210, 211, 213, 216, 222
DKK-1, 66, 77
drugs, 8, 84, 92, 174, 210, 213
duodenum, 153, 154, 155, 191, 193

E

edema, 36, 101, 154
encephalomyelitis, 138, 140, 211, 217, 218, 228, 229
encoding, 70, 116, 129, 157
endothelial cells, 13, 21, 22, 36, 38, 40, 142, 211
endothelium, 37, 42, 44
endotypes, 101, 103, 110
end-stage lung disease, 116
enthesitis, 61, 62, 64, 68, 69, 70, 71, 72, 73, 78
environment, 23, 44, 50, 84, 87, 110, 216, 221, 224, 225, 227
environmental factors, 32, 39, 85, 100, 101, 157, 158, 173, 189
enzymes, 122, 189, 190, 191, 196, 197
eosinophilic infiltration, 102
eosinophilic inflammation, 124

eosinophils, 40, 85, 90, 91, 101, 103, 105, 106, 107, 112
epithelial cells, 93, 104, 106, 119, 125, 142, 207, 210, 211, 214, 217
epithelium, 87, 102, 103, 131, 211
erosion, 13, 14, 16, 66, 69, 77
esophagus, 153, 155
etiology, 62, 138, 139, 158, 173
Europe, 100, 156, 165, 168, 173
evidence, 6, 32, 35, 36, 40, 68, 69, 86, 96, 102, 123, 136, 141, 164, 173, 180, 183, 187, 191, 200, 205, 211, 212, 213, 223
experimental autoimmune encephalomyelitis, 140, 211, 217, 229
exposure, 3, 84, 100, 182, 183, 188
extracellular matrix deposition, 32, 33

F

fibroblast growth factor, 125, 135
fibroblast proliferation, 37
fibroblasts, 23, 28, 33, 36, 38, 40, 43, 51, 59, 77, 78, 104, 106, 125
fibrosis, 32, 33, 34, 36, 37, 38, 39, 40, 42, 44, 46, 48, 51, 52, 103, 107, 115, 116, 118, 124, 127, 128, 129, 130, 131, 132, 133, 134, 135, 136
fingolimod, 145, 146, 149
fluid, 13, 15, 19, 24, 25, 63, 64, 69, 70, 71, 76, 77, 79, 102, 113, 121, 131, 144, 209
focal inflammation, 138
formation, 63, 65, 66, 67, 72, 77, 88, 105, 138, 143, 154, 191, 197, 212
fractures, 77, 161, 196
functional activation, 51

G

gastrointestinal tract, 33, 116, 152, 153, 155, 196

Index

gene expression, 42, 46, 85, 105, 185, 210, 216, 223, 224, 226

genes, 34, 63, 74, 104, 105, 125, 146, 157, 158, 189, 210, 223

genetic factors, 70, 86, 139, 158, 197

genetic predisposition, 85, 86, 173, 192

genetics, 167, 168

genome, 63, 69, 70, 215

genotype, 101, 165, 199

genotyping, 70, 74

glutamate, 43, 190

gluten, 187, 188, 189, 190, 191, 193, 194, 195, 196, 197, 198, 199, 200, 201, 202, 203, 204

gluten enteropathy, 187, 188, 189, 195, 204

GM-CSF, 2, 15, 37, 87, 142, 144, 211

Golimumab, 71, 175, 176

gross domestic product, 156

growth, 37, 56, 59, 116, 117, 127, 160, 161, 164, 192, 218

guidelines, 126, 127, 136, 176

H

healing, 185, 210, 212, 216

health, 8, 58, 100, 125, 136, 215

heterogeneity, 2, 8, 10, 16, 18, 20, 50, 58, 100, 108, 109, 213, 215

histological examination, 193, 194, 197

histology, 124, 162, 163, 194, 197, 203

history, 94, 101, 119, 161, 165

HLA, 63, 64, 69, 70, 73, 75, 187, 189, 190, 191, 194, 199, 202

HLA-B27, 63, 70, 73, 75

homeostasis, 34, 42, 44, 46, 55, 76, 88, 91, 104, 157, 174, 183, 185, 207, 221, 222, 225

host, 1, 4, 6, 7, 10, 110, 118, 123, 125, 128

human, 2, 5, 8, 9, 11, 12, 13, 14, 17, 18, 19, 20, 21, 22, 26, 27, 28, 36, 54, 55, 56, 68, 78, 79, 103, 105, 111, 112, 124, 133, 135, 141, 144, 189, 202, 207, 211, 213, 215, 217, 218, 227, 228

humoral immunity, 52, 140

hyperemia, 154

hypersensitivity, 84, 134, 187, 188, 194, 197, 206

hypothesis, 45, 84, 94, 108, 120, 224

I

IBD, 102, 151, 152, 153, 155, 156, 157, 158, 159, 160, 161, 162, 163, 164, 165, 166, 167, 168, 169, 172, 173, 174, 181, 182, 183, 185, 209, 212, 213, 216, 222, 223, 224, 225

IBD-unclassified, 153, 155, 156, 162

idiopathic, 47, 152

IFN, 8, 9, 15, 17, 19, 26, 28, 35, 59, 76, 85, 89, 90, 95, 106, 122, 141, 144, 148, 191, 207, 208, 217

IFN-β, 148

IFNγ, 2, 3, 17, 91, 140, 141, 144, 187, 199

IFN-γ, 35, 76, 85, 89, 90, 95, 144, 191

IFNγ+Th17 cells, 17

IgE antibodies, 89

IgE-mediated, 85, 206

IL-13, 35, 85, 87, 89, 91, 105, 106, 107, 140

IL-17B, 37, 40, 49, 59

IL-17E, 37, 40, 49, 51, 59, 105

IL-17F, 2, 12, 36, 37, 40, 49, 62, 63, 68, 88, 89, 92, 96, 103, 107, 113, 122, 141, 143, 144

IL-22, 2, 37, 38, 39, 44, 52, 63, 64, 65, 68, 71, 76, 80, 88, 89, 90, 96, 107, 130, 138, 141, 142, 146, 159, 191, 202, 208, 211, 212, 213, 219

IL-23, 3, 6, 19, 28, 39, 41, 43, 52, 56, 57, 63, 64, 65, 68, 69, 70, 71, 72, 73, 74, 78, 88, 103, 105, 111, 112, 113, 120, 122, 141, 145, 159, 169, 208, 212, 213, 218, 222, 223

238 *Index*

IL-4, 35, 36, 71, 85, 87, 89, 91, 105, 106, 124, 140, 141
IL-5, 35, 85, 87, 90, 105, 106, 107, 113, 124, 140, 141
IL-6, 6, 11, 12, 13, 14, 15, 18, 23, 36, 37, 39, 41, 42, 43, 49, 50, 52, 56, 57, 63, 68, 69, 88, 105, 106, 120, 121, 123, 124, 126, 134, 138, 141, 142, 147, 159, 169, 174, 191, 206, 208, 222, 223, 224, 225
IL-8, 13, 14, 15, 36, 38, 39, 62, 69, 88, 103, 106, 124, 125
immune reaction, 117, 174
immune regulation, 41, 50, 111
immune response, 5, 7, 27, 31, 34, 36, 42, 84, 85, 87, 89, 90, 91, 101, 102, 107, 112, 119, 127, 143, 158, 159, 187, 190, 200, 208, 218, 222, 224
immune system, 32, 33, 35, 85, 104, 118, 125, 139, 158, 173, 199
immunity, 1, 2, 4, 5, 7, 9, 39, 40, 50, 88, 95, 100, 105, 106, 108, 112, 113, 116, 118, 119, 129, 173, 191, 201, 202, 222
immunodeficiency, 50, 157, 194
immunoglobulin, 34, 63, 87
immunomodulatory, 122, 123, 124, 131, 138, 145
immunomodulatory therapy, 138, 145
immunosuppressants, 145, 175
immunosuppression, 44, 54, 181
immunotherapy, 110, 131, 148, 199
in vitro, 5, 15, 16, 28, 77, 124, 134
in vivo, 21, 43, 95, 112, 132, 185
indeterminate colitis, 155, 166
individuals, 4, 16, 32, 38, 40, 54, 66, 101, 119, 139, 158, 173, 190, 192, 207, 223
induction, 9, 12, 51, 55, 58, 59, 72, 89, 104, 116, 121, 140, 181, 207, 217, 219
INF, 23, 124, 159, 160
infection, 4, 5, 6, 7, 57, 117, 118, 119, 121, 122, 125, 127, 128, 130, 131, 135, 194
infectious agents, 100, 158, 162, 221
inflammatory arthritis, 25, 26, 59, 61, 62

Inflammatory Bowel Disease (IBD), 102, 124, 151, 152, 153, 155, 156, 157, 158, 159, 160, 161, 162, 163, 164, 165, 166, 167, 168, 169, 170, 172, 173, 174, 181, 182, 183, 184, 185, 186, 209, 212, 213, 216, 217, 218, 219, 222, 223, 224, 225, 226, 227, 229
inflammatory cells, 36, 37, 85, 86, 87, 90, 117, 211, 227
inflammatory disease, 2, 11, 12, 43, 55, 58, 85, 87, 104, 132, 139, 185, 216, 229
inflammatory responses, 51, 116, 190, 207
inhibition, 7, 16, 20, 22, 25, 26, 28, 39, 41, 44, 56, 66, 67, 81, 90, 123, 133, 147, 217, 225, 228
inhibitor, 13, 18, 19, 26, 66, 68, 71
initiation, 36, 102, 140, 142, 149, 174, 175, 206, 217
innate lymphoid cells, 1, 6, 9, 10, 62, 76, 77, 78, 79, 88
integrity, 125, 135, 142, 212
interferon, 4, 8, 27, 69, 71, 134, 143, 145, 146, 149
interleukin-17, 21, 22, 23, 24, 25, 26, 27, 28, 48, 50, 51, 58, 76, 80, 96, 134, 201, 214
interstitial lung disease, 45, 47, 48
intervention, 106, 128, 148
intestinal homeostasis, 174, 183
intestinal tumorigenesis, 213
intestine, 154, 157, 160, 165, 198
iron, 161, 162, 192, 195
issues, 20, 170

J

joint damage, 70, 78
joint destruction, 13, 15, 19
joints, 12, 13, 14, 23, 63, 65, 68, 69, 70, 72, 74, 75, 78, 161, 209

Index

L

lead, 4, 19, 36, 71, 84, 85, 86, 89, 105, 121, 122, 123, 127, 140, 142, 158, 180, 184, 194, 197, 207, 212, 221, 224

lesions, 39, 51, 54, 55, 139, 141, 142, 151, 154, 160, 197, 208, 211

leukocytes, 105, 211

leukotrienes, 86, 87

life expectancy, 116

ligand, 13, 15, 34, 46, 67, 68, 69, 89, 159, 211

liver, 52, 161, 166, 184, 194, 195

lung disease, 116, 123, 127, 128, 130, 134

lung function, 87, 100, 109, 111, 120, 121, 123, 125, 126, 127, 129

lung infection, 4, 127

lung transplantation, 134

lupus, 45, 107

lupus erythematosus, 45

lymph, 2, 87, 119, 130, 142

lymph node, 2, 87, 119, 130, 142

lymphocytes, 1, 2, 35, 40, 46, 47, 58, 85, 87, 88, 91, 101, 103, 106, 107, 108, 113, 119, 120, 124, 130, 140, 142, 143, 144, 145, 146, 172, 174, 178, 190, 193, 215, 221, 222, 224

lymphoid, 1, 5, 6, 9, 10, 16, 62, 76, 77, 78, 79, 88, 101, 160, 225

lymphoid tissue, 5, 225

M

macrolides, 116, 122, 123, 124, 125, 132, 133, 134

macrophage inflammatory protein-3 α, 14

macrophages, 4, 14, 40, 59, 88, 105, 106, 120, 123, 124, 140, 141, 142, 143, 208, 218

magnetic resonance, 77, 141, 153

magnetic resonance imaging, 77, 141

majority, 69, 156, 188, 210, 223

malabsorption, 189, 192, 195, 203

mast cells, 40, 62, 64, 70, 71, 72, 74, 76, 85, 90, 103, 106, 107

matrix metalloproteinase, 14, 20, 38, 67, 140

measurement, 40, 145, 190, 198

mechanical stress, 67, 68

medical, 130, 160, 231

medication, 91, 194

medicine, 83, 111, 153, 231

memory, 17, 26, 34, 38, 46, 56, 69, 79, 130, 141, 144, 185, 223

meta-analysis, 18, 24, 26, 27, 132, 202

metabolism, 67, 69, 122

metalloproteinase, 14, 20, 67

MHC, 70, 73, 140, 207

mice, 3, 4, 5, 6, 9, 24, 38, 51, 59, 64, 76, 90, 104, 122, 124, 129, 134, 140, 213, 228

microvascular aberrations, 33

migration, 14, 25, 38, 42, 44, 68, 88, 94, 102, 111, 142, 211

models, 2, 4, 13, 15, 18, 22, 36, 38, 63, 68, 71, 89, 90, 102, 116, 120, 121, 207, 209, 210, 212, 213, 222

molecules, 34, 37, 47, 69, 123, 140, 142, 143, 160, 174, 190, 191

monoclonal antibodies, 26, 174, 183

monoclonal antibody, 27, 66, 80, 213

morbidity, 4, 116, 131

mortality, 4, 116, 131

motif, 15, 51, 68, 159

mRNA, 13, 15, 19, 207, 213, 223

mucin, 116, 121, 125

mucosa, 2, 3, 79, 85, 86, 87, 90, 92, 130, 151, 154, 159, 160, 161, 169, 173, 183, 185, 187, 190, 191, 192, 193, 195, 197, 199, 201, 209, 210, 216, 222, 223, 224, 226

mucosal secretion, 87

mucous membrane, 6, 193

mucoviscidosis, 116

mucus, 117, 121, 128

Multiple Sclerosis (MS), 50, 52, 54, 77, 80, 93, 102, 107, 125, 137, 138, 139, 140, 141, 142, 143, 144, 145, 146, 147, 148, 149, 166, 184, 206, 209, 210, 211, 229

muscles, 68, 192

mutations, 115, 116, 157, 158

myelin, 139, 140, 141, 143

myofibroblasts, 38, 42, 44

N

nasal ovalbumin, 90

nasal provocation, 87

nasopharyngeal colonization, 4

necrosis, 20, 21, 185, 216

nervous system, 138, 144, 147, 198, 205, 206, 210, 215, 217

neurodegeneration, 138, 139

neurodegenerative diseases, 139

neutrophil recruitment, 207

neutrophilic airway inflammation, 104

neutrophilic inflammation, 84, 89, 103, 116, 117, 120, 123, 207

neutrophils, 4, 38, 62, 64, 68, 70, 72, 90, 102, 115, 117, 121, 123, 124, 142, 154, 173, 197, 206, 207

NOD2/CARD15 mutation, 157

nonradiographic axial SpA, 62

Notch signaling, 43

O

obstruction, 52, 86, 99, 100, 101, 106, 108

obstructive lung disease, 114, 131

oligodendrocytes, 139, 142, 143

organ, 33, 39, 211

organism, 2, 101, 118, 174, 221, 222

organs, 2, 31, 32, 42, 44, 62

osteoclast, 12, 13, 19, 69, 79

osteoclastogenesis, 11, 12, 13, 14, 19, 20, 21, 22, 28, 62, 71, 72, 77, 79

osteoporosis, 161, 192

overproduction, 38, 49

oxidative stress, 142, 211

P

P. aeruginosa, 115, 117, 118, 120, 121, 122, 125, 126

pain, 160, 161, 189, 192, 196

pathogenesis, 2, 4, 11, 12, 16, 20, 26, 31, 32, 33, 35, 36, 39, 40, 43, 44, 45, 47, 48, 49, 50, 52, 60, 62, 63, 67, 70, 72, 73, 78, 84, 88, 90, 92, 103, 107, 108, 111, 128, 138, 139, 142, 145, 147, 151, 158, 159, 160, 164, 168, 184, 187, 191, 196, 197, 199, 201, 202, 205, 206, 208, 209, 221, 225

pathogens, 3, 85, 102, 104, 115, 120, 127, 129, 174

pathology, 6, 101, 148, 160, 212

pathophysiological, 86, 92, 101

pathophysiology, 61, 139, 163

pathway, 13, 18, 25, 26, 28, 43, 51, 61, 62, 64, 66, 68, 69, 70, 73, 74, 75, 78, 84, 92, 130, 221

pathways, 6, 7, 21, 23, 31, 32, 36, 56, 86, 100, 106, 108, 113, 116, 121, 127, 159, 168, 174, 202, 205, 206, 228

pediatric IBD, 151, 152, 153, 156, 157, 160, 161, 163, 165, 166, 167, 168, 169, 170

pemphigus, 208, 214

pemphigus vulgaris, 208, 214

peptide, 20, 73, 193, 200

peptides, 104, 140, 189, 190, 199, 201

peripheral blood, 5, 16, 17, 25, 26, 38, 42, 46, 47, 50, 54, 55, 60, 65, 69, 71, 76, 88, 91, 99, 105, 108, 109, 120, 121, 138, 142, 172, 175, 176, 177, 178, 180, 184, 209, 218, 224

Index

241

peripheral blood mononuclear cell, 5, 16, 25, 46

permeability, 87, 125, 159, 173, 190, 197

Peyer patches, 3

phagocytosis, 124, 128

pharmacokinetics, 132, 133, 136

phenotype, 2, 3, 35, 55, 92, 101, 104, 106, 119, 121, 131, 144, 151, 159, 163, 164, 165, 208, 211

phenotypes, 32, 49, 55, 101, 102, 104, 109, 111, 114, 122, 143, 144, 154

phosphorylation, 39, 52, 89, 146

physical activity, 100

placebo, 27, 80, 81, 126, 132

plaque, 138, 143

plasticity, 16, 17, 20, 26, 42, 55, 186, 191, 200, 210, 211, 217

pneumococcal carriage, 5

pneumococcal whole-cell vaccine, 5

pneumococci, 2, 4, 5

polarization, 16, 221, 224

population, 56, 59, 79, 85, 109, 113, 120, 146, 156, 157, 166, 167, 177, 180, 202

preservation, 124, 221

prevention, 4, 6, 132, 209, 225

prognosis, 163, 198, 213

pro-inflammatory, 1, 2, 12, 37, 38, 39, 43, 63, 88, 102, 117, 141, 142, 144, 159, 191, 206, 207, 209, 222

proliferation, 5, 20, 34, 36, 38, 39, 41, 46, 77, 90, 124, 183, 212, 225

prostaglandin, 13, 78, 134

protection, 1, 2, 4, 5, 6, 7, 66, 77, 85, 110, 207

proteins, 78, 140, 142, 159, 188, 207, 208, 210, 211

psoriasis, 68, 70, 71, 72, 107, 124, 146, 197, 199, 209

psoriatic arthritis, 62, 68, 74, 75, 77, 78, 79, 80, 81

pulmonary diseases, 100, 103, 106, 107, 108, 109, 132, 134

Q

quality of life, 61, 62, 85, 125, 147, 203

R

race, 156, 173

RANKL, 13, 14, 28, 67, 69, 70, 79

reactions, 84, 126

reactive arthritis, 62, 73, 76

receptor, 15, 16, 18, 21, 22, 25, 27, 33, 34, 39, 46, 49, 59, 63, 64, 66, 67, 68, 69, 79, 103, 104, 110, 111, 112, 134, 141, 145, 146, 159, 183, 210, 218

receptors, 23, 24, 37, 45, 51, 87, 89, 105, 133, 146, 148, 175, 226

recognition, 87, 152, 158, 190, 199

recommendations, 162, 166

recovery, 183, 193, 195

regeneration, 64, 76

regulatory T cells, 3, 25, 45, 50, 51, 53, 54, 55, 56, 57, 75, 102, 104, 130, 134, 149, 169, 185, 186, 202, 216, 217, 227, 228, 229

rejection, 107, 120, 125

relapses, 141, 142, 147

relevance, 65, 74, 135, 226

remission, 71, 172, 177, 178, 182, 193

researchers, 38, 39, 43, 91, 108, 123

resistance, 125, 129, 138, 146, 151, 165, 199

respiratory tract, 83, 85, 86, 92, 103, 106, 107, 116, 133

response, 4, 7, 16, 18, 21, 23, 25, 27, 34, 40, 59, 63, 69, 75, 81, 84, 85, 86, 88, 89, 90, 92, 95, 96, 101, 103, 105, 106, 107, 108, 113, 117, 118, 122, 124, 125, 127, 129, 139, 143, 145, 172, 173, 177, 182, 183, 184, 187, 197, 199, 206, 218

retinoic acid orphan receptor, 104

reversible bronchial obstruction, 101

242 *Index*

Rheumatoid arthritis, 6, 10, 11, 12, 20, 21, 22, 23, 24, 25, 26, 27, 28, 29, 32, 33, 36, 50, 53, 102, 107, 124, 185, 209, 215, 216, 217, 228, 229

rhinitis, 83, 84, 85, 90, 91, 93, 94, 95, 96, 97, 103, 104, 105, 106, 112, 113, 206

risk, 70, 74, 81, 86, 100, 106, 108, 113, 119, 121, 126, 131, 138, 143, 146, 147, 156, 157, 158, 188, 189, 195, 196, 212, 213

RORγt, 41, 43, 88, 159, 183

S

S. aureus, 3

S. pneumoniae, 4, 6

sacroiliitis, 62, 70

safety, 6, 18, 26, 29, 74, 80, 199

salivary glands, 17, 26

scleroderma, 38, 46, 47, 51, 55

sclerosis, 31, 32, 40, 45, 46, 47, 48, 49, 51, 52, 53, 54, 55, 56, 57, 58, 59, 60, 138, 147, 148, 209, 210

secrete, 1, 36, 37, 42, 44, 105, 107, 141, 142, 173, 191

secretion, 1, 2, 7, 14, 15, 34, 37, 38, 39, 54, 62, 85, 87, 107, 117, 124, 125, 129, 130, 131, 134, 140, 142, 173, 175, 191, 192

Secukinumab, 18, 27, 28, 65, 66, 71, 72, 74, 78, 79, 80, 81, 199, 204

sensitivity, 22, 34, 126, 190, 192, 194, 201

sensitization, 84, 101, 131, 198

serology, 192, 194, 197

serum, 15, 25, 35, 39, 40, 46, 47, 50, 51, 58, 64, 66, 71, 90, 91, 108, 113, 123, 126, 133, 141, 159, 162, 183, 190, 194, 203, 208, 209, 214, 222

severe asthma, 96, 100, 102, 106, 108, 109, 110, 113, 207

short-term memory, 212, 218

showing, 16, 183, 191

signaling pathway, 24, 28, 38, 39, 48, 51, 77, 159, 191, 226

skin, 2, 22, 31, 32, 33, 34, 36, 38, 39, 42, 44, 45, 46, 48, 49, 51, 54, 55, 62, 69, 72, 79, 112, 116, 134, 161, 188, 197, 205, 206, 208, 214

skin diseases, 206, 208, 209, 214

skin lesions, 39, 51, 54, 55, 197, 208

SLE, 32, 33, 42, 47, 209

sleep disturbances, 100

small intestine, 162, 172, 187, 188, 189, 190, 197, 201

smooth muscle, 38, 42, 51, 87, 101, 102, 103, 106, 111, 116, 121, 125, 135, 207

smooth muscle cells, 38, 42, 51, 103, 106, 116, 121, 125, 135

species, 12, 107, 117, 144

spondylitis, 62

Spondyloarthritis, 61, 62, 74, 75, 76, 77, 78, 79, 81

sputum, 108, 125, 134, 207

stabilization, 63, 125

steatorrhea, 189, 192

stimulation, 5, 7, 14, 68, 71, 89, 115, 119, 120, 141, 190

stromal cells, 23, 24, 48

structure, 37, 49, 154

submucosa, 106, 108, 115, 120

substrate, 143, 190

suppression, 42, 43, 53, 90, 134, 173, 222, 226, 228

surface protection, 2

survival, 34, 41, 122, 131, 132, 183, 207, 219

susceptibility, 9, 14, 18, 23, 24, 34, 39, 46, 52, 63, 70, 73, 75, 121, 122, 129, 189

symptoms, 18, 69, 79, 80, 85, 86, 87, 90, 96, 99, 100, 101, 108, 109, 116, 117, 138, 140, 143, 146, 160, 161, 189, 190, 192, 196, 198, 203, 210, 222

synaptic plasticity, 212, 218

Index

243

syndrome, 17, 26, 36, 87, 100, 101, 102, 110, 138, 143, 144, 158, 192, 194, 195, 196

synovial endothelial cells, 13, 21

synovial fluid, 13, 15, 19, 21, 24, 25, 63, 64, 69, 70, 71, 76, 77, 79, 209

synovial tissue, 12, 20, 69

synoviocytes, 12, 13, 15, 21, 22, 23, 28, 69

synovitis, 11, 12, 15, 19, 26, 70, 72, 73, 74, 81

synthesis, 13, 14, 38, 40, 42, 44, 87, 120, 142

systemic lupus erythematosus, 32, 33, 47, 53, 58, 209

systemic sclerosis, 31, 32, 40, 45, 46, 47, 48, 49, 51, 52, 53, 54, 55, 56, 57, 58, 59, 60, 209

T

T cell receptor, 226

T cells, 3, 4, 8, 9, 13, 15, 18, 19, 21, 22, 27, 28, 36, 38, 39, 40, 41, 43, 45, 46, 50, 52, 53, 54, 55, 56, 62, 63, 64, 68, 69, 70, 72, 74, 75, 76, 78, 79, 88, 95, 96, 102, 103, 104, 112, 119, 120, 130, 134, 140, 141, 142, 143, 146, 149, 160, 177, 181, 183, 185,186, 190, 191, 201, 202, 205, 206, 210, 211, 214, 215, 216, 217, 219, 223, 224, 227, 228, 229

T effector cells, 172

T follicular helper, 3

T lymphocytes, 1, 2, 17, 26, 31, 35, 47, 60, 84, 87, 88, 91, 107, 177, 183, 185, 191, 216, 222

T regulatory cells, 1, 2, 9, 53, 54, 104, 175, 185, 207, 216, 219, 221, 222, 224

target, 17, 37, 43, 89, 103, 160, 197, 211

testing, 57, 189, 193, 194, 197, 198

TGF, 16, 36, 41, 42, 44, 52, 55, 66, 88, 89, 95, 112, 141, 143, 159, 191, 228

TGFb, 5, 89, 222

Th cells, 17, 26, 35, 39, 40, 89, 91, 103,

Th17 cytokines, 13, 22, 43, 74, 75, 112, 116, 122, 169, 202

Th17/Treg balance, 5, 16, 42, 43, 209

Th2 immune response, 84, 87, 89, 90, 91, 101, 102

Th22 cells, 71, 142, 146, 148, 202, 208

T-helper cell, 104, 119, 140, 206, 222, 225

therapeutic approaches, 43, 106

therapeutic effects, 105, 228

therapy, 17, 18, 20, 25, 27, 28, 43, 50, 52, 53, 69, 71, 73, 75, 80, 92, 101, 103, 108, 113, 116, 126, 127, 133, 136, 138, 145, 146, 147, 149, 151, 163, 165, 172, 174, 175, 176, 177, 178, 179, 180, 181, 182, 183, 184, 185, 187, 195, 196, 200, 213, 214, 216, 217, 219, 225, 228

thrombocytopenia, 42, 57

thrombocytosis, 161, 162

tissue, 8, 21, 32, 36, 37, 43, 55, 64, 68, 78, 88, 94, 101, 103, 104, 105, 107, 118, 123, 124, 127, 173, 197, 201, 205, 206, 207, 209, 212, 223, 224, 225

tissue inflammation, 37, 205, 206, 207

TNF, 6, 8, 11, 12, 13, 14, 15, 16, 18, 19, 22, 24, 25, 27, 34, 39, 59, 63, 65, 66, 68, 69, 71, 72, 75, 79, 80, 81, 85, 89, 91, 123, 142, 159, 160, 171, 185, 206, 213, 214, 215, 216, 219, 226

TNF-alpha, 214, 219

TNF-α, 3, 6, 11, 12, 13, 14, 15, 75, 22, 24, 59, 79, 89, 91, 119, 123, 138, 140, 142, 143, 159, 160, 172, 173, 174, 175, 176, 177, 178, 180, 181, 182, 183, 184, 185, 216, 229

toxic effect, 198

Tr-1 cells, 3

transcription, 8, 9, 18, 25, 37, 41, 43, 55, 63, 64, 70, 88, 104, 146, 159, 177, 180, 190, 215, 223, 224, 225

transcription factors, 8, 104, 159

244 *Index*

transducer, 37, 64, 159
transforming growth factor, 66, 69, 159
transplantation, 120, 125
treatment, 3, 7, 25, 27, 29, 45, 66, 68, 72, 73, 78, 80, 81, 90, 104, 106, 108, 110, 123, 126, 133, 136, 138, 145, 146, 147, 148, 172, 174, 175, 177, 178, 179, 180, 181, 182, 183, 184, 185, 187, 188, 195, 196, 198, 199, 200, 213, 216, 226
Tregs, 3, 5, 16, 57, 104, 171, 172, 174, 175, 177, 178, 179, 180, 181, 182, 183, 184, 191, 209, 210, 222, 223, 224, 225, 228
trial, 27, 71, 81, 126, 132, 135, 199, 204
tuberculosis, 107, 162, 175
tumor, 7, 11, 12, 24, 25, 27, 28, 34, 79, 81, 159, 205, 206, 213, 217, 228
tumor necrosis factor, 11, 12, 24, 25, 27, 28, 34, 79, 81, 159, 217, 228
tumorigenesis, 213, 218

U

ulcerative colitis, 107, 152, 153, 155, 160, 166, 168, 172, 184, 227
ulcerative colitis (UC), 107, 152, 153, 154, 155, 156, 157, 158, 159, 160, 162, 163, 164, 166, 168, 169, 170, 171, 172, 175, 176, 177, 178, 179, 180, 181, 182, 184, 227
upper respiratory tract, 83, 86

urban, 93, 131
urbanization, 84, 93
Ustekinumab, 29, 70, 72, 80, 213, 219

V

vaccine, 1, 2, 5, 7, 8, 9, 187, 188, 198, 199, 200, 204
validation, 170
vascular endothelial cells activation, 36
vascular endothelial growth factor, 13, 22, 125, 135
vascular endothelial growth factor (VEGF), 13
viruses, 86, 129, 139
visceral organ fibrosis, 33
vitamin B1, 161, 192
vitamin B12, 161, 192
vitamin B12 deficiency, 161
vitamins, 139, 192

W

weight loss, 160, 161, 189, 192, 196
Wnt, 22, 66, 71, 77
worldwide, 4, 100, 138, 145, 153

Related Nova Publications

ANTIPHOSPHOLIPID ANTIBODIES (APLA): TYPES AND FUNCTIONS IN HEALTH AND DISEASE

EDITOR: Luke E. Ward

SERIES: Immunology and Immune System Disorders

BOOK DESCRIPTION: The opening chapter of *Antiphospholipid Antibodies (APLA): Types and Functions in Health and Disease* is focused on the modern immunoassays for the determination of aPL in biological fluids.

SOFTCOVER ISBN: 978-1-53613-971-6
RETAIL PRICE: $82

OLD AND NOVEL HUMORAL BIOMARKERS OF AUTOIMMUNE MYASTHENIA GRAVIS

AUTHORS: Giovanni Luca Masala, Davide G. Corda, M.D., Giovanni A. Deiana, Giannina Arru, and GianPietro Sechi, M.D.

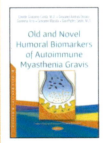

SERIES: Immunology and Immune System Disorders

BOOK DESCRIPTION: Autoimmune Myasthenia Gravis (MG) is mediated by pathogenic autoantibodies to components of the postsynaptic muscle endplate at the neuromuscular junction. Due to the clinical heterogeneity of the disease, there is a great need for objective biomarkers for diagnostic as well as therapeutic purposes.

SOFTCOVER ISBN: 978-1-53613-836-8
RETAIL PRICE: $95

To see a complete list of Nova publications, please visit our website at www.novapublishers.com

Related Nova Publications

HELPER T CELLS: TYPES, FUNCTIONS AND NEW RESEARCH

EDITOR: Brando Boudewijn

SERIES: Immunology and Immune System Disorders

BOOK DESCRIPTION: *Helper T Cells: Types, Functions and New Research* presents current research in the Tfh cell research field with a special focus on the maintenance of TFH cells and their fate once the immune response has resolved.

SOFTCOVER ISBN: 978-1-53613-070-6
RETAIL PRICE: $82

CHRONIC GRANULOMATOUS DISEASE: GENETICS, BIOLOGY AND CLINICAL MANAGEMENT

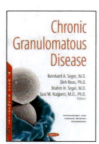

AUTHORS: Reinhard A. Seger, Dirk Roos, Brahm H. Segal and Taco W. Kuijpers

SERIES: Immunology and Immune System Disorders

BOOK DESCRIPTION: This is the first e-book on Chronic Granulomatous Disease (CGD). This book is meant for everyone involved in the diagnosis, treatment or guidance of patients with this disease, as well as for the patients and their parents/caretakers, investigators and students experiencing this disease.

ONLINE ISBN: 978-1-53612-498-9
RETAIL PRICE: $0

To see a complete list of Nova publications, please visit our website at www.novapublishers.com